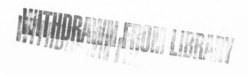

The Silicone Breast Implant Controversy:

What Women Need to Know

by
Frank B. Vasey, M.D.
and
Josh Feldstein

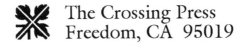 The Crossing Press
Freedom, CA 95019

ABA8227

To Paulette
and Bonnie

This book is intended to provide information about breast implants and implant-related symptoms. This book is not intended to be, and does not constitute, medical advice.

The views expressed in this book have been formed by discussions with the authors' colleagues, plastic and general surgeons, and other physicians and medical industry experts. They reflect opinions of the authors.

The names and identifying facts of the patients in the case studies have been changed to protect their identity.

Copyright © 1993 by Frank B. Vasey and Josh Feldstein
Cover art and design by AnneMarie Arnold
Printed in the U.S.A.

Library of Congress Cataloging-in-Publication Data

Vasey, Frank B.
    The silicone breast implant controversy: what women
    need to know / by Frank B. Vasey and Josh Feldstein.
        p. cm.
    Includes index.
    ISBN 0-89594-609-2 (paper). —ISBN 0-89594-610-6 (cloth)
    1. Breast implants—Complications. 2. Silicone—Toxicology.
    3. Consumer education.   I. Feldstein, Josh.   II. Title.
RD539.8.V38 1993   93-29670
618.1'9059—dc20   CIP

Acknowledgments

A heartfelt thanks to our wives, Paulette Vasey and Bonnie Nulty Feldstein, whose support, wisdom, hard work, and love helped make this book possible.

Special thanks to Ed Decker and Linda Carbone for their expert editorial assistance—and all matters literary and emotional.

Dr. Vasey would also like to acknowledge the assistance and support of the entire Division of Rheumatology at the University of South Florida College of Medicine. Helen Barnwell, Kathy Walls, and Kim Harding answered calls from around the country. Deborah Havice, R.N., assisted in seeing patients and honing the concept of a silicone-induced illness. Fellow rheumatologists on the faculty, Bernard F. Germain, M.D., Mitchel J. Seleznick, M.D., Tomas S. Bocanegra, M.D., and Paul Bridgeford, M.D., in private practice—each and all contributed to the care of women with breast implants and rheumatic disease. Alvin Wells, Ph.D., studied the immunology of the breast capsule. The medical school administration, Roy H. Behnke, M.D., Marvin R. Dunn, M.D., and Ronald P. Kaufman, M.D., offered unfaltering support from the beginning.

Most importantly, Luis R. Espinoza, M.D., an esteemed colleague and co-worker of almost 20 years in two medical centers, deserves credit for being the first in our group to recognize this emerging medical condition.

A word of thanks as well to all the plastic surgeons who helped us with the book and the care of patients. Further, our appreciation to Megan Svensen, Lisa Benoit, John Singer, and Joe Diamond for their help during the research and creation of the manuscript.

Warmest thanks are extended to Audrey Penn for her unending commitment and love throughout the writing and editing process.

And, finally, a deep and sincere word of acknowledgment to all of Dr. Vasey's patients, the dozens of brave women who poured out their stories of pain for this book, and those many hundreds of others who inspired, taught, cajoled, harassed, supported, and sustained the entire USF rheumatology team during the long and continuing struggle for the recognition of silicone-related problems.

Table of Contents

Foreword

As the host of a nationally syndicated TV talk show, I made the difficult decision to go public with my silicone breast implant ordeal and told my story to *People* magazine in February 1992. This personal nightmare spanned eleven years and included five sets of implants. I was tremendously relieved at the thought of unburdening myself of what had been a well-guarded secret, and I also felt that I had a responsibility to come forward. I encourage other celebrities to do the same.

Once the article was published, I was inundated with calls and letters from other women who had implants. They were scared, they were sick, and they were desperate for information. Their deep need made me realize how little I really knew about breast implants.

I consider myself to be a well-informed individual. I read newspapers and magazines, watch television news programs, and listen to the radio. But these news sources offered scant information about breast implants and silicone disease. Sure, there had been some splashes of coverage about various lawsuits, as well as Food and Drug Administration (FDA) investigations. But there had been many unclear and conflicting reports about the safety or danger of silicone. When your health is at stake and there seems to be nothing but unanswered questions, fear is bound to take hold. With the publication of *The Silicone Breast Implant Controversy: What Women Need to Know*, we *finally* have a resource—a place to go for answers and for help.

Many of the women who wrote to me explained that they had decided on implants because they "just didn't feel like a woman." Having had implants for those same wrong reasons, I certainly understand this attitude. Now I am horrified at the notion that so many of us thought two gel-filled prostheses would be the missing ingredient to our womanhood. It calls into question so many things, perhaps the saddest being the cultural pressure for perfection in women's bodies, which hundreds of thousands of us are willing to attempt to reach through surgery. Many of us succumbed to our poor self-image with breast implants only to face the trauma of our "perfect" breasts, which we fantasized about for so long, becoming hard and desensitized. Suddenly we become fixated on our chests in a whole new way. "I'd do anything to get my old body back," I've heard over and over. "I just want the chemical making me sick out as quickly as possible!" Our picture of our new sexiness is shattered when we can't allow ourselves to be seen or touched from the waist up. I empathize with women who are driven to barbaric measures because they are sick

1

and unable to find a plastic surgeon to remove their implants, or those who simply can't afford to have it done. Some have even taken razor blades to their own chests to rid themselves of the source of the pain. I had one woman write and tell me that she actually stuck a pin into her implant in an attempt to "psychologically relieve the pressure and the pain." These acts of desperation should never have happened. Becoming informed is our first priority.

Among the women looking for answers are the ones who have been doubly traumatized, having had breast implants due to a mastectomy. It is my belief that these women have a right to make an informed choice and, with the help of this book, that decision may at last be made based on good information.

In my own search for help—adding insult to injury—I found most plastic surgeons to be unsympathetic, patronizing, and arrogant. (A case in point is a barbaric, insulting poem that was in a letter to the editor in the July 1992 issue of *Journal of Plastic and Reconstructive Surgery* about "women who are aug'd." Read it if you dare.) It also amazes me that many physicians to this day continue to deny that silicone-induced disease exists. My guess is that many are all too aware of its danger but are afraid to say so for fear of their colleagues' reaction.

I recently had a plastic surgeon on my show who, before we went on the air, said that he thought silicone implants were terribly dangerous and that he wouldn't implant them even with a gun held to his head. When I posed a question about the implants while we were on the air, however, his response was that he thought they were just fine and that he'd still be putting them in if it weren't for the FDA's moratorium. I just sat there in disbelief. Another plastic surgeon wrote to me when the *People* story first came out, saying he thought I must be "hysterical for scaring people the way you did." I don't know if it's because most of the doctors are male and breast implant recipients are female, but quite a few women believe that there would have been a lot more questions regarding the dangers of implants—not to mention appropriate testing—if *men* were sporting them.

Like so many women who opted to "improve" themselves and their self-image cosmetically with breast implants, I felt shame about my body. There is so much pressure on women to look a certain way by the constant exposure to pictures, ads, and magazine covers showing the idealized sexy woman. Ironically, a lot of these models have been liposuctioned or implanted themselves, not to mention that fashion photos are commonly retouched! Nonetheless, the average woman knows her husband or boyfriend sees such images and may feel she must do something if she doesn't measure up. Yet how can we expect to live up to these images *when they are not real to begin with?*

Again, like many other women, my poor self-image began at home. I don't blame my parents, but while I was growing up I was always getting comments about being flat-chested, mostly from my father. If only my parents could have commented more on the things that come from the *inside*, I believe it may have helped me develop a far healthier, balanced perspective of myself and my body.

There is nothing wrong with a concern for appearance, but we must not let our images of ourselves be shaped and dictated by the outside world. I got my implants because it was my perception that large breasts would make me more attractive. Now I know that my beauty was always there. I just found it the hard way.

Luckily, the surgeon who finally removed my implants referred me to a psychotherapist to help me sort out all the emotions I confronted after my lengthy ordeal. Talking to a therapist helped me immeasurably in dealing with the traumas I had endured, and enabled me to confront the self-esteem problems that had made me choose implants in the first place. I think that any woman dealing with silicone disease should seek the help of a trained counselor.

Despite the progress I have been fortunate enough to have made, not a day goes by that I don't wonder how my exposure to silicone is affecting my health. With every ache, every pain, the question arises: Is it the silicone? My surgeon took out what he could, but it's not possible for all of the silicone to be removed. I don't expect ever to lose that fear.

My silicone breast implant problems forced me to take responsibility for my health in a way I had never done before. My hope is that with the help of *The Silicone Breast Implant Controversy*, the pain and suffering of hundreds of thousands of women and their families will be diminished and, more important, avoided by women in the future. I passionately support and admire the courage and dedication of its authors in communicating the much-needed, much-deserved truth that all of us who have fallen prey to silicone deserve to know. Frank Vasey and Josh Feldstein's book should be considered essential reading for *any* woman who has come into contact with silicone!

— Jenny Jones

Preface

"Women greatly overestimate society's tastes in breast size," noted Dr. J. Kevin Thompson in a recent psychology study. What's more, "women's beliefs about men's preferences are wrong, and this incorrect belief may be the reason why women opt for breast implants: trying to achieve a cultural ideal they believe others have."[1] Other research, noted Dr. Jennifer Brenner, a Professor of Psychology at Brandeis University, found that "female models are 9% taller and 16% thinner than average women—an unrealistic ideal of beauty to emulate, which contributes to low self-esteem."[2] Another study, noted Kristen Golden, coordinator of a Ms. Foundation for Women effort to promote women's issues, found that "up to age 11, girls are very straightforward and confident. They trust their own experience and say what they think. [But] by age 12, they're beginning to get mixed messages from their families, the media and society . . . that they're supposed to be quiet, nice, thin, and preferably blonde. I think if we stopped lying . . . to our girls, they would be in much better shape."[3]

Clearly, feelings of physical inferiority serve to create a ripe environment for women to embrace "changes" such as breast implantation. A study published several years ago based on research with 2,000 women found that they were less satisfied than men with their appearance and were more critical of their bodies.[4] Another study observed that of 1,100 women queried, 48 percent said they would be more attractive if they lost 20 pounds.[5] The cultural stage has thus been set for women to be unhappy about their physical appearance.

In recent decades, there has been a growing acceptance of high-tech means to alter nature's endowment. But lest anyone think that alteration of a woman's shape to achieve some ideal is new, consider the whalebone corsets of the nineteenth century that forced women into unnatural hourglass shapes, often at the expense of their digestive health (though probably few studies were done to prove it). Consider, too, the breast-lifting, cleavage-forming dresses of centuries past.

The choice to alter one's body is a personal one, and many women are delighted with the results they have achieved through breast augmentation with silicone and saline implants. It nevertheless remains a strange fact that we live in a society that makes women compare their bodies to a perfect—and often unattainable—ideal, taking their self-worth and self-identity from their appearance only, some going so far as to put themselves through difficult and expensive ordeals to achieve such goals.

5

In our sexually stereotyped society, it's little wonder, then, that so many women have willingly undergone surgery to achieve the perfect image of femininity. Of over 640,000 cosmetic surgical procedures in 1990, breast augmentation ranked second only to liposuction.[6] Can you imagine the same number of men requesting plastic surgeons to enlarge their penises or to have their buttocks tightened? More important, can you imagine men having to wait nearly 30 years before serious problems affecting their health were finally investigated and brought out into the open?

Frank B. Vasey, M.D., was alerted in the mid-1980s to the possibility that immune response to silicone breast implants could cause rheumatic disease. His opinion was influenced by specific reports from a handful of other rheumatologists, as well as daily interactions with Luis Espinoza, M.D., at the University of South Florida College of Medicine. By 1989, Dr. Vasey's clinical observations of his patients convinced him that an important women's public health issue had been almost completely ignored by medicine, industry, and government: silicone implants could lead to serious health problems in susceptible individuals.

In December 1990, when the late Congressman Ted Weiss (D-NY) requested Vasey's testimony before the Government Operations subcommittee, his medical observations drew widespread press coverage. This media exposure subsequently led hundreds of symptomatic women with silicone implants from around the country to contact Vasey for advice and treatment. To date, he has personally treated nearly 500 women with breast implants who are suffering from rheumatic disease.

This book has been written in an attempt to clarify the complex issues regarding breast implants, the immune system, rheumatic disease, and the governmental, industry-related, and societal elements that have led to this health care debacle. The ultimate decision to have breast implants placed or removed is critical to both a woman's psychological and physiological health. Women making either decision must be as fully informed as possible. This is the book's major concern.

Additionally, this book is intended not only for women who have silicone breast implants—those who feel well, and those who do not—but for their partners, families, and friends as well. It is also for women considering implants. It is the authors' hope that this work will be viewed as a contribution to the medical community as a whole, especially to those health care providers who encounter and attempt to help women suffering from silicone-related medical problems.

6

At the same time, our book is not intended to resolve the silicone breast implant controversy. Only well-designed, large-scale epidemiologic studies will serve ultimately to convince physicians and, in particular, plastic surgeons of the existence of what we call silicone-associated connective tissue disease. Nor has this book been written to sensationalize the medical issues or to scare people. The overwhelming majority of the estimated 1 million women with implants will most probably never develop any kind of illness from their prostheses. Exactly what percentage of them will become ill remains to be determined.

Originally, silicone was used in breast implants because silicone itself was believed to be inert when in contact with body tissues. Over the years, silicone devices have included hypodermic needles, cardiac pacemakers, artificial joints, testicular implants, artificial heart valves—and silicone has even been used in a form known as simethicone for over-the-counter (OTC) digestive aids and infant formulas. Considering that 8 of 10 women who have received implants have done so for augmentation, it's no surprise that cosmetic rather than medical factors were primary in the development of the silicone breast implant.

For years, all types of implants were positioned by both implant manufacturers and plastic surgeons as harmless, inert objects. These include silicone gel–filled implants with a smooth or textured outer silicone envelope; inflatable saline-filled implants in silicone envelopes; and double lumen silicone implants, which have a silicone balloon within another silicone balloon, one filled with gel and the other saline. Questions about implant-related side effects—other than capsular contracture (the accumulation of fibrous tissue surrounding the implant)—were very often brushed aside, and most patients were led to believe they wouldn't even know the implants were there. However, the fact—noted in the fine print of some package inserts—that no implant was *ever* warranted to be a lifelong resident in a woman's body did not seem to be made clear, or clear enough.

The Silicone Breast Implant Controversy is organized to provide the reader in Part I with a complete spectrum of current medical information about silicone-associated connective tissue disease, how the implants affect the body, and the specific clinical manifestations of the illness in the patient and her immune system. Part II offers a historical background—from the early 1960s to the present—regarding the development of the implant controversy, as well as the often complex interactions among the FDA, industry, and the doctors involved. Part III delineates the practical considerations every woman faced with an implantation or explantation decision must know in order for her to make the best possible health care decision. In the appendix, the book provides general information on breast surgery, as well as sources for additional data on silicone disease from numerous support organizations.

Though silicone-associated connective tissue disease has received much attention, the majority of women with implants, as well as their physicians and surgeons, do not yet hold a clear picture of what silicone disease is, how it develops, how to diagnose it, and what to do about it. Worse, the very existence of the disease is still being contested by many physicians. It is our hope that *The Silicone Breast Implant Controversy: What Women Need to Know* will replace confusion with clarity, hopelessness with direction, and fear with reason.

Part I: Silicone

Chapter 1

The Difficulties in Diagnosing Silicone-Induced Disease

When she was 34, Rachel had her breasts enlarged with silicone implants. She had been completely flat-chested all her life, was never able to get clothes to fit her, and was especially self-conscious in a bathing suit. A petite woman at 100 pounds, even with her implants her bust size was only 34 A or B, depending on the bra. But after having had a hysterectomy at age 29, she needed an emotional and physical lift, and breast augmentation surgery seemed like a good idea.

As a registered nurse who worked in a general surgery ward, Rachel had seen over 50 women come in for silicone breast implants. In every case, the surgery went smoothly and the patient left thrilled with her new body and her new self-esteem. "The more I saw, the more I liked the idea," she said. The short-term, postoperative follow-up results looked excellent in every case she had observed over a three-year period, the only complication being an occasional hardening of breast tissue over the implant. But Rachel had looked into that, and had been well assured by the plastic surgeon that it was "easy to resolve."

So, with her husband's blessing, she scheduled herself for surgery. Everything went well, and she was extremely pleased with her new look. Motivated by her changed appearance, she soon began to exercise regularly on Nautilus equipment and to take an hour-long run three or four times a week. Her new physique improved her self-confidence, made her feel "so much better" about herself, and had a positive effect on her sex life with her husband. For 10 years, life was good.

Then, beginning at age 44, Rachel slowly became aware of a few annoying symptoms. Her eyes were becoming drier and drier, as was her mouth. For the first time in her life, she began to experience fluid retention. Sometimes she found herself short of breath—nothing too serious, just an occasional wheeze when she exhaled.

She assumed it was perhaps a bit too much exercise. After all, she was getting a little older, and maybe all the running and workouts were getting to be too strenuous. When she began to have difficulty breathing at night—lying in bed, or just sitting and relaxing—she started to get scared. Sometimes she felt the wheezing and shortness of breath for no reason at all; other times it appeared to be exercise-induced. She made an appointment with her doctor to check it out. He diagnosed asthma and instructed Rachel to use a Ventolin inhaler several times a day to keep her lung passages open. But the sprays didn't seem to help. In fact, the asthma worsened almost on a daily basis. She went back to the doctor, who gave her first the steroidal spray Vanceril and later several other inhalers to see whether any could offer relief. None did. He then put her on a large dose of the oral bronchodilator Theodur, which gave her uncontrollable shaking and spells of vomiting. Alarmingly, not only did her breathing problems get more serious, but she began to experience terrible chest pains, at times so bad it felt as though her chest cavity were being crushed. One night the pain got so unbearable that Rachel went to the emergency room, convinced that she was having a heart attack.

The physicians at the hospital also suspected a heart attack. They began monitoring Rachel's heart on an electrocardiogram (EKG), which noted that her heart's electrical waves were abnormal. They studied her heart muscle, valves, and arteries by ultrasound and cardiac catheterization. They gave her a stress test. The diagnosis? It wasn't a heart attack, but the doctors didn't know what it was. They labeled it a panic attack. Rachel, who knew it was no panic attack, was nevertheless released from the hospital, placed on several medications for her heart—including beta blockers and nitroglycerin (which gave her terrible headaches), given a new inhaler and bronchodilator for her breathing—and sent home. Her life had become agonizing, scary, depressing. She felt completely isolated.

As time went on, Rachel became sicker. Virtually every joint in her body gave her great pain. Swallowing also became difficult. The chest pain and pressure continued—always bad, sometimes terrible. Though she hated the idea of living on pills, she took her medications religiously, even though they didn't seem to be doing any good; she was afraid *not* to take them. She had escalated to an astounding 40 puffs a day on three different inhalers, and her breathing still continued to worsen.

Next her lymph nodes began to swell, the pain coursing down her arms and through her chest wall. It became more and more difficult to breathe. Back to the hospital she went, getting more and more desperate. Further testing was done: another computer axial tomography (CAT) scan, more X-rays, tests for adrenal tumors, complete endocrine and pulmonary workups, repeated urinalyses, and tests that inject dye into the arteries of the kidneys, causing extremely painful side effects. Again, the tests showed nothing conclusive.

Back home, Rachel felt new pains in her lower abdomen that went straight down to her groin. Her gallbladder began to hurt, too. Back to the doctors, more tests, more seemingly normal results, more items added to the growing list of symptoms. Worst of all, Rachel began to realize that the doctors were running out of answers. Eventually her general practitioner sent her to a specialist. After two weeks, he had nothing to offer Rachel either. No one seemed to know what to do. She mentioned to her physicians that the problems might be connected to her implants, but none of them acknowledged the possibility, noting that purely anecdotal information and inconclusive lab tests were not enough to go on.

She began to wonder, very seriously, whether she was losing her mind. Were her problems all in her head? In the midst of these grave self-doubts,

Rachel began to fear that no one believed her. Only she knew, absolutely knew, that something was horribly wrong with her body.

During all these months of frustration and pain, Rachel somehow continued to work at the hospital. At least work offered some release from her isolation. But her concentration and memory were failing her. When the other nurses noticed her obvious mental lapses, she tried to joke about them, calling them "mentalpause." She fought hard not to lose hope that she might recover.

For quite a while she had noticed a steady diminution in her sexual feelings, and now her desire for sex seemed to be disappearing altogether. Ever since she had her implants placed, more than a decade before, she had been aware of a loss of sensitivity in the outer half of her right breast. Now the numbness spread to her left nipple as well. But the worst was not over. Rachel now developed hypertension, which failed to respond to one medication after another. She had by this point become so chronically exhausted that she felt as if her "power supply had shorted out." Poor concentration continued to affect her work, as she wandered off midstream on irrelevant tangents. She began to have night sweats, she was pulled from sleep due to the frequent need to urinate, she lost her appetite, and eventually she stopped sleeping. She was "a wreck, a total wreck," she told anyone she could confide in. Then a series of inexplicable rashes erupted all over her face and body. She started to develop tremors and muscle weakness in her arms, hands, and legs. She felt constantly nauseous, as though she were "always pregnant." She developed a polyp on her gallbladder. She lost 20 pounds in 60 days. And then she hit bottom. "I wanted to die," she said. "I didn't care if I died."

Rachel decided to have her implants removed. In the first five months after removal (*explantation*), some things, like her breathing and lung problems, got a little better, but her muscle and joint pain did not improve. "There are more questions than answers at this point," she said with resignation. "Nobody knows the long-term effects of silicone disease. Will I ever be normal again? I ask myself every day whether I'll ever get well, or if this disease will be a way of life for me."

Like every other woman who becomes ill from silicone disease and opts to have her implants removed, Rachel had to confront a range of emotional scars. Often "mistaken for a child" before she had implants because of a lack of breast tissue, she explained that she "now looks like a ten-year-old boy."

"I am a nurse," she continued. "I know what illness is. Not every woman who gets implants becomes sick—many are lucky and never do—but those who do, like me, go from doctor to doctor and from test to test and get nowhere because there are so few doctors who understand silicone disease." Countless other patients confirm this experience. Many have wiped out their savings in the process due to a lack of insurance coverage, or due to their existing insurance excluding them. "Some women I know have been told by their doctor that they simply didn't want to see them again," she added.

Silicone disease, due to its varied nature, is an illness that requires a fitting together of a constellation of signs and symptoms. Unfortunately, a single lab test to confirm silicone disease, such as the one used to confirm strep throat, does not yet exist. Hence few physicians have been able to identify the disease in their patients, and therefore have instituted a long chain of blind testing and trial medications.

To make diagnostic matters even more complex, great skill is required to conduct a pathological evaluation with a standard laboratory microscope in order to catch silicone particles in tissue. Far more sophisticated and expensive technologies, such as high-powered electron microscopy/X-ray dispersive analysis, can be used to identify silicone in the body, but this is far beyond what is generally available in most doctors' offices.

Additionally, the early signs of silicone disease are often nonspecific, the types of symptoms that can occur in anyone. Later, as the illness proceeds, its symptoms often evolve into conditions that appear similar to nonsilicone-induced rheumatic diseases, such as rheumatoid arthritis, lupus, and scleroderma. This combination of nonspecific and rheumatic symptoms, all of which appear to be similar to other illnesses, makes misdiagnosis easy. What's more, a physician who sees only an occasional silicone disease patient may easily misdiagnose her symptoms as a rheumatic ailment not linked to her implants. But should the physician develop an interest in silicone disease and see hundreds of patients with the same patterns, the constellation of silicone-induced signs and symptoms soon becomes clear.

It is important to understand that modern specialization and subspecialization in medicine lead physicians to develop exceptional skill in one area and little in others. It is probably true that many of the plastic surgeons who insert breast implants stay away from any involvement in the postoperative, implant-induced medical complications of their patients, and that most rheumatologists are not trained or experienced in plastic surgery procedures.

Simply put, surgeons tend to focus on a single problem or area of the body. They will take a generally healthy patient, address a specific surgical problem—an infected gallbladder, for example—remove it, and be finished. Medical problems that might occur following surgery would normally be referred to an internist, family practitioner, or other medical specialist, because that's not what the surgeon handles. Internal medicine, on the other hand—and rheumatology is a subspecialty of internal medicine—is oriented toward the assessment of all the body systems and how these systems integrate.

Unlike surgeons, rheumatologists cannot often solve problems quickly or completely. Very often they must work with a patient day after day to fight an ongoing battle. And that is precisely the nature of treating silicone-induced disease. As in virtually all rheumatic and autoimmune illnesses, the goal is to do everything possible to maximize the patient's health. Often, that's the maximum success a rheumatologist can achieve. This work is clearly less dramatic than that of the surgeon. Patients who suspect they may be getting ill from silicone need to recognize the inherent complexity of this medical question as well as the training and orientation of their physician.

Chapter 2

The Medical Facts About Silicone Implants

They need all this proof, they say. How many of us do they need for proof? Women are dying from them . . . .

Following breast reconstruction for fibrocystic breast disease (benign breast tumors or cysts), Laura got silicone implants in 1984 at the age of 35. A few months later, she became extremely fatigued and developed flulike symptoms. She found it difficult to get through a day of work as a medical office manager. Her doctor told her she had some sort of connective tissue disease, but all the tests came back negative.

As the years passed new symptoms appeared. She returned to her doctor and received a new diagnosis of some kind of virus. She began to have dizzy spells and her hair started falling out. She developed mouth ulcers, rashes, joint pain, and muscle pain. Finally, she went to the University of South Florida's Department of Rheumatology, where she was diagnosed as having silicone-associated connective tissue disease. It was recommended that she have the implants removed. "I originally thought Dr. Vasey was crazy," said Laura. Then she began talking with other women who had had similar problems and quickly realized that Dr. Vasey could be right.

Laura didn't want her plastic surgeon touching her again, so she had a general surgeon remove her implants in 1989. The pathology report showed that both of her implants had ruptured at the seam, leaking silicone into her body. The surgeon had to remove the lymph nodes from both of Laura's underarms in an effort to get the silicone out.

Recovery has been slow, although at least the rashes have cleared up. Laura has to use a cane now and often finds herself breaking into tears or throwing things in anger when she is home alone. She used to be a PTA president and was involved in many different personal and professional activities; now she needs all her energy just to get through each day. She maintains that she would have committed suicide if it weren't for her two children.

The Unfolding of a Disease

Much evidence on how silicone can cause various autoimmune and rheumatic disorders has come to light in recent years. However, long before recent media exposés, the medical establishment had been warned about the dangers of silicone.

Reports in leading medical journals, results from manufacturers' preclinical (animal) experiments, and scores of complaints brought into doctors' offices by women with implant-related problems—all have contributed to our current knowledge of how these prosthetic devices can ravage a woman's health and immune system and even in some cases send her into suicidal depression, total disability, or emotional breakdown. Yet it took virtually three decades for regulatory officials at the FDA to blow the whistle. The reasons it took so long can be attributed to mistaken diagnoses, blind or willful denials, information gaps, and massive bureaucratic foot-dragging.

The first women believed to have their breasts enlarged with silicone were Japanese, possibly in the mid- to late 1940s. In these cases, liquid silicone gel, as well as paraffin and other substances, were injected by syringe directly into the breasts. Many of these women were prostitutes who had discovered that American servicemen preferred women with larger busts than were common in Japanese women. Concern about their health was apparently a very low priority.

Beginning in the 1950s, physicians in the United States began using injections of liquid silicone as well, in addition to implanting sponges directly into women's breasts. The practice was continued for years. According to a report in the *American Journal of Nursing*, it was finally banned by the FDA due to a wide range of "disastrous" complications, including infections from improperly sterilized silicone materials and patient injuries and deaths.[7] All other silicone injection procedures used by plastic surgeons and dermatologists for alterations such as lip enhancement and the smoothing of facial wrinkles have also since been completely halted by the FDA.

The search for a healthier and safer way to introduce silicone into the female breast for the purpose of physical enhancement led to a major advance in 1961. That year, Drs. Thomas Cronin and Frank Gerow, who later joined implant manufacturer Dow Corning, first combined rubbery and liquid silicone to create a soft but firm gel. They enclosed the gel in a silicone-rubber envelope. The implant was surgically placed in a Houston woman in 1962, and the era of surgical breast enhancement began.

Silicone-gel implants have been widely used since 1976. Saline-filled silicone envelope devices have also been implanted, but less frequently; they have the same silicone shell as gel implants but are filled with a sterile saltwater solution. (Since the FDA's moratorium on gel-filled implants in 1992, these have been the only legal implant prostheses unless a woman is enrolled in a clinical trial. However, saline implants are now also under FDA investigation.)

"Some people have argued that [silicone implants] have to be proven unsafe before the FDA can act to protect patients against their use," stated FDA Commissioner David Kessler in April 1992. "This is *not* so. The burden of proof is an *affirmative* one, and it rests with the manufacturer. We know more about the life span of automobile tires than we do about the longevity of breast implants. And we do not know whether there is any link between implants and immune-related disorders and other systemic diseases. Until these basic questions are satisfactorily answered, the FDA cannot approve these devices." These words sent the implant industry reeling.

Plastic surgeons and others may argue that the data implicating silicone implants definitively in the cause of serious illness is not as yet strong enough. But based on the suffering of patients, as well as the *burden of proving safety*, according to the FDA (which, sadly, was articulated 20 years too late), it is our opinion that silicone implants are dangerous and unproven. In fact, according to a Medical Devices Bulletin issued by the FDA, following testimony provided by a panel of medical experts in late 1991 prior to Dr. Kessler's decision, the FDA noted that data from *all four* manufacturers "did not provide reasonable assurance of safety" in the areas of:

- Implant rupture.
- Gel bleed and the potential of silicone migration (throughout the body).
- Chemical information on silicone and silicone gel.
- Toxicity regarding the immune system, cancer, and birth defects.
- Tumor detection.
- Psychological issues.

To make matters worse, implant manufacturers had known since 1976—when the medical device law statute was passed, "grandfathering" medical devices (including implants) already on the market (that is, excluding them from providing additional safety data)—that they would one day be called upon to provide the FDA with additional scientific evidence of safety. Well, more than 15 years later, as demonstrated by the FDA panel's findings, the manufacturers still had not done their safety data homework. The obvious question is, did they know something they wanted to keep secret?

Was Evidence About Silicone Dangers Available to Doctors?

Silicone had been successfully used for many years in a host of medical devices, with virtually no bad publicity regarding biological or autoimmune incompatibility. So the medical establishment embraced the practice of placing foreign silicone objects into women's bodies *before* those objects were rigorously tested for safety.

In addition to erroneous assumptions about safety, six other factors have delayed the medical community's full knowledge of silicone's potentially dangerous nature.

1. Lack of access to foreign studies.

Numerous articles published in Japanese medical journals in the early 1960s documented cases of rheumatic disease, including a threefold increase in scleroderma (a fibrotic thickening of skin and vital organs) in women who had been injected many years earlier for breast enlargement. Unfortunately, due to the language difficulty and cultural lags, findings of these types—which often referred to the illness as "human adjuvant disease" (as noted in Drs. Kumagai and Shiokawa's 1979 "Arthritis and Rheumatism" publication concerning four patients with scleroderma)—did not begin to appear in North American and British journals until the late 1970s.[8] (Additionally, among the 128 pieces of general medical implant literature on public file in the Dockets Management Department of Health and Human Services of the FDA as of May 1990, of those publications that discuss gel leakage or migration in any way, only about one dozen were published prior to 1980.) Even when these findings were made available, however, some American physicians and the FDA attributed the problems to the use of inferior-quality silicone, paraffin, and other substances—not the medical-grade silicone used in American implants. While this was a legitimate criticism of the Japanese reports, it might also have been a convenient way for plastic surgeons to avoid taking a closer look into the lucrative and growing implant business. After all, the FDA relied on plastic surgeons to advise them of problems.

2. Implants were not evaluated for safety by the FDA.

Before the disclosures of industry and the media forced the issue to a head, patients assumed that silicone-gel implants had long ago been deemed safe. Interviews with University of Southern Florida (USF) patients and others indicate that few plastic surgeons reviewed possible systemic risks in any significant detail and that, unless specifically requested, they had not provided patients with the package inserts that came with the implants. As of January 1982, however, silicone implants had been only *preliminarily* (not officially) placed in Class III by the FDA—which meant the devices would be evaluated and regulated to assure safety and effectiveness—given that the FDA believed the devices posed "a potentially unreasonable risk of injury."[9]

Still, safety data from manufacturers—due to the 1976 grandfather statute—did not require research findings to be submitted for FDA review. Implants slipped through an unusual loophole.

After the publication of the Japanese findings in English-language journals in the late 1970s, only a limited number of other reports of silicone-related illnesses appeared in the medical literature, including one paper by B. F. Uretsky et al. in 1979 in the *Annals of Plastic Surgery*.[10] This article described a woman who nearly died of kidney failure before her implants were removed. But the publication of these reports failed to spur significant action. Around the same time, other papers were published, also apparently without much attention, in such publications as *The Journal of Aesthetic Plastic Surgery*, *The American Journal of Clinical Pathology*, *The British Journal of Plastic Surgery*, *Plastic and Reconstructive Surgery*, *The Journal of the American Medical Association*, *Arthritis & Rheumatism*, and *The Archives of Pathology and Laboratory Medicine*.

Then in January 1984 an article appeared in *Arthritis & Rheumatism*, written by two well-respected rheumatologists in Pittsburgh, Tom Medsger and Gerald Rodnan.[11] It described 18 patients who had signs of rheumatic disease and silicone implants. It was this report that focused the attention of the University of South Florida Division of Rheumatology on the issue.

Between 1984 and 1988, rheumatologists at the USF began to see many more implant recipients with signs and symptoms of rheumatic illness; yet only an occasional paper on the subject was published in the medical literature. It is generally believed that many surgeons and physicians who did look into the correlation of rheumatic illness and silicone implants found it to be inconsequential. Nobody thought silicone implants could cause rheumatic diseases, nor were they viewed as a potential public health problem. As a result, not until June 1988—26 years after the first implant—did the FDA issue a final regulation to classify breast implants as potentially dangerous, confirming them as a Class III device, thus *requiring* more stringent regulation. It was not until early 1992 that the FDA finally called for a complete moratorium on and an investigation into silicone-gel implants.

3. Company communications lacking.

In 1984, the FDA began the Medical Device Reporting (MDR) Program, which required manufacturers to report to the FDA all failures of devices noted by surgeons. However, the information gathered was not directly disseminated to patients via product literature, and so a critical link in the communication chain broke down. It was not until the following year that Dow Corning (the largest of the implant manufacturers until dropping out of the estimated $500-million-a-year marketplace in 1992) began noting the risk of "immunological problems" on their package inserts. And as recently as 1991, in a 14-page patient information booklet, only one short paragraph near the end of Dow's brochure bothered to address autoimmune disease at all.

Not surprisingly, after the implant controversy began to escalate, Dow Corning began running an "educational" advertising series, inviting concerned patients to call a hotline for the "facts" on implant safety.[12] On December 30, 1991, the FDA sent a warning letter to Dow Corning stating that some of the information provided to women over the company's toll-free information line was "false or was used in a confusing or misleading context." The FDA cited "verbal statements made by Dow Corning's hotline staff that overstated the safety of their implants or minimized known or suspected side effects. [The] FDA documented these false or misleading statements, including assertions that breast implants are 100% safe, [and that] the FDA advisory panel (which met on November 12–14, 1991) said that breast implants were safe, that silicone cannot migrate to other organs in the body, and that breast implants have never been linked to autoimmune or connective tissue diseases." Finally, the memo stated that "the FDA believes that Dow Corning's hotline is falsely reassuring women of the safety of breast implants when studies have not fully shown the frequency of known adverse effects, nor whether potential long-term effects such as autoimmune disease can be linked to the implants."[13]

4. Follow-up studies by plastic surgeons on patients receiving silicone implants ended too soon.

Because plastic surgeons only occasionally track their patients' recovery beyond a short time after surgery—more than a year or two is uncommon—many of those surgeons who used silicone-gel implants never knew that some of their patients developed silicone-related disorders later on.

Additionally, in all the years that silicone implants have been used, the American Society of Plastic and Reconstructive Surgeons (the primary professional organization for board-certified plastic surgeons) completed few surveys to ascertain patient satisfaction with implants. Based on their findings in one specific survey, they claimed—and aggressively publicized—a higher than 90 percent happiness level, according to their promotional materials.[14] The data was obtained via a questionnaire mailed to women one, two, and three years following implantation of their prostheses. In one USF study, however, the average woman developed the onset of silicone disease symptoms about 4 1/2 years after implantation. Thus, the findings of the Plastic Surgeon's Society did not address the medical condition of silicone recipients at the more critical times of 5 to 10 years postoperatively and were therefore incomplete. In contrast, a long-term prospective study is still sorely needed to demonstrate implants' safety and their effects on the health of recipients.

5. Autoimmune disorders are often outside the expertise and general interest of plastic surgeons.

Many of the reports about silicone-related disorders were published in medical journals outside the field of plastic surgery. It is unlikely that a plastic surgeon would read a rheumatology abstract or keep up with the latest developments in immune disorders.

But in 1991 and 1992, a small number of investigators presented their findings concerning the potential connection between silicone-gel implants and illness at the annual meeting of the American Society of Plastic and Reconstructive Surgery (ASPRS). The response was often skepticism or outright rejection—not surprising, given that plastic surgeons who do augmentation procedures see happy patients shortly after the operation, not seriously ill women years later.

6. Doctors may not realize that their patients have implants.

Until very recently, most women who have become ill with a variety of seemingly unrelated disorders never dreamed that their problems might be caused by their implants. As a result, few thought it worth mentioning to their doctors that they had them. Our interviews have shown, in fact, that soon after getting them, many women view their implants as part of their bodies and so may be unlikely to think of them as disease-causing objects. Other women may feel embarrassed discussing their implants with a physician; some never tell their internist, obstetrician, gynecologist, spouse, or lover that they had breast augmentation surgery. And because scarring is often minimal, depending upon the incision site, even a physical examination may not enable a doctor to spot an implantation.

Today, although most physicians require new patients to indicate previous surgeries, some continue to ignore this history for one reason or another, further complicating the silicone disease connection. (One *beneficial* side effect of the publicity on this issue, however, is that there is now an increased likelihood that women will more readily tell their physicians they have implants.)

Silicone Migration and Leakage:
The Starting Point for Disease

Implant manufacturers have maintained for many years that silicone implants are safe and inert. Yet simply placing an implant on a paper napkin will produce an observable absorption of gel on the paper within hours. While this "bleeding" effect does not, in itself, prove toxicity, it certainly raises reasonable doubts about silicone safely remaining within the implant. This "bleeding," moreover, occurs in all implant recipients, and is the first—and fastest—means by which the body can be exposed to silicone.

It is hypothesized that because the gel and the outer envelope are both made from the same material—elemental silicon and oxygen—it is possible for the gel to slip through the microscopic pores in the outer envelope due to pressure (from wearing a bra or carrying a grocery bag against the chest, for example) or even due to the simple force of gravity over time.

I have talked to so many doctors who know absolutely nothing about it . . . .

After having her polyurethane foam–coated implants explanted due to many years of problems—including gallbladder removal, pneumonia, hospitalizations, irritable bowel syndrome, memory loss, and joint pain—Nina had a mammogram that was interpreted by three different doctors as indicating breast cancer. She claims her plastic surgeon did a "rushed botch job" in removing the implants (her primary-care physician literally had "to scream at the surgeon on the phone" to get him to do the explantation in the first place), leaving behind large amounts of silicone gel that had escaped into her body. Nina's heart sank when she was told she needed mastectomies on both breasts. In desperation, she got a fourth opinion and was told that what looked like cancerous growths on her mammogram may have been gel residue from the implant. She was operated on, and a voluminous amount of leaked gel was removed. No sign of cancer was found in either breast. Recovery from silicone disease remains quite slow for her, however.

Then, of course, there is the risk of leakage due to rupture, which is virtually equivalent (physiologically) to gel injection. This can occur regardless of whether the implant is placed directly under the breast tissue (between the mammary glands and the chest muscle) or under the chest muscle against the chest wall. Many factors have been shown to cause rupture—from a cut during a breast biopsy, to the bite of an infant, to the pressure exerted by a shoulder strap during an automobile accident. Highly active women who ski or windsurf may also put too much stress on their implants, causing the seams to burst open and gel to leak into the body. Wherever the silicone goes, scarring, swelling, and inflammation may occur.

Rheumatic Reactions to Silicone: A New Disease?

While many autoimmune/rheumatic diseases appear troublingly similar in patients both with and without silicone implants, some implant recipients differ in the manifestation of their disease in key ways—thus supporting the notion of a specific syndrome dependent on silicone exposure.

Studies and clinical observations have shown that rheumatic/autoimmune disorders caused by silicone exposure may differ in some women from the classic rheumatic disorders, and that these women tend to improve with removal of the implants. Implant patients also experience frequent muscle pain and tenderness in the anterior chest wall around the prostheses and commonly describe an unusual burning character to the pain.

Rheumatic conditions affect the body's joints, muscles, and connective tissue (which hold together the structure of the body), including tendons and cartilage. Silicone exposure can affect the entire musculoskeletal system in numerous and serious ways.

Under normal circumstances, inflammation is an important component of the healing process: it creates an environment conducive to tissue repair and to the elimination of bacterial invaders. In the case of rheumatic ailments, this same healing process turns injurious, adversely affecting healthy joints, muscles, and connective tissues adjacent to the areas of inflammation. Should these inflammatory conditions last for a prolonged period of time, the localized rheumatic effects may become systemic, appearing in all parts of the body. And since exposure to silicone in women with implants is most often measured in years, such long-term exposure can induce chronic inflammation.

Some women with implants show atypical combinations of clinical findings. When the manifestations of silicone-associated connective tissue disease are severe and widespread, it comprises a syndrome not typically encountered by physicians: severe chronic fatigue causing a patient to sleep as much as 10 hours but awakening exhausted; fibromyalgia pain (musculoskeletal pain and stiffness) with diffusely tender muscular trigger zones; joint pain, generally without swelling, but occasionally with mild swelling of wrists and ankles; swollen lymph nodes (lymphadenopathy) in the underarm and neck that wax and wane; and mysterious burning/crawling sensations indicative of peripheral nerve malfunction. In a woman with silicone disease, all this occurs with a borderline positive antinuclear antibody test (ANA), but in the absence of a "butterfly" facial rash on the cheeks or kidney disease (which would suggest instead that the patient has systemic lupus erythematosus).

The presence of antinuclear antibodies in a woman's blood, while typical of systemic lupus erythematosus, is not unique to that disorder. In fact, most women with a positive ANA do not have lupus. The test really serves as an indication of immune stimulation occurring in a variety of clinical situations ranging from chronic infectious hepatitis to cancer, to multiple chronic inflammatory rheumatic diseases. Research in this area continues with several new publications. Richard Silver, M.D., a rheumatologist from Charleston, found elemental silicon in the skin, joint lining, and lung tissue of three women with breast implants using X-ray dispersive analysis and electron microscopy. Henry Claman, M.D., an immunologist from Denver, reported the prevalence of antinuclear antibodies in groups of women with and without breast implants. While normal women without implants had a 5 percent prevalence of a positive ANA, asymptomatic women with implants had a 30 percent prevalence of positive ANA. What's more, symptomatic women with implants but without defined connective tissue disease had a 50 percent prevalence. Finally, women with implants and defined connective tissue disease showed a 90 percent prevalence.

Additionally, Eric Gershwin, M.D., and co-workers in rheumatology from the University of California at Davis, have recently described anti-collagen antibodies in women with breast implants.

While none of these observations are definitive, they all support the concept that silicone may diffuse widely throughout the body and is a stimulant to the immune system.

Turning next to *fibromyalgia*, when rheumatologists use this term, they mean tender knots of muscle (trigger zones) caused by a combination of injury, strain, and overuse, as well as a light, nonrestorative sleep pattern in a tense, anxious/compulsive individual resulting in chronic pain. Immune malfunction is not thought by most rheumatologists to play a central role. In fibromyalgia patients, there is pain and tenderness in muscles and *around* joints, but not typically *in* joints—a clinical manifestation seen far more often only in silicone patients.

Additional evidence supporting the association of silicone and connective tissue disease comes from observations of women with traumatic breast implant rupture. Our research in a small group of women who were in good health while the implants were in place has shown that shortly following implant rupture, these women developed the typical muscle pain, joint pain, and swelling of rheumatic disease, which improved or stabilized once the rupture was recognized and the implants removed. In addition, women known to have experienced a silicone-gel breast implant rupture at a certain time (following a specific traumatic event, for example) have developed chronic fatigue, and muscle and joint pain, shortly thereafter.

How can physicians and patients determine that silicone, rather than other coincidental factors, is causing an immune response and clinical illness? While there is no way to be absolutely certain, USF rheumatologists have observed that *a common constellation of symptoms shows up in a high percentage of women with implants who develop problems.* As mentioned earlier, these symptoms appear on average a little more than four years after implantation, but the range extends from immediately after surgery to 22 years later. Here are the most common symptoms of silicone disease documented thus far, in order of frequency:

- Chronic fatigue.
- Inflammation and muscle pain (myalgia), initially in the anterior chest, back, and neck (pain may radiate beyond these areas); muscles are weak, tender, stiff, and sensitive to the touch.
- Joint pain and swelling.
- Swollen lymph nodes (from pea-sized to lima bean–sized lumps) in the chest, neck, underarms, and groin (junction of legs and abdomen).
- Low-grade fever (100° to 101°).
- Gastrointestinal symptoms, including cramping and abdominal pain.

Other symptoms include:
- Night sweats.
- Memory loss.
- Dry eyes and mouth.
- Headache.
- Rashes.
- Difficulty swallowing.

- Bladder problems, including interstitial cystitis (chronic inflammation of the bladder) and frequent urination in the absence of infection.
- Sinus irritation.
- Numbness and altered sensation in the body.
- Skin tightening, either locally or bodywide.
- Lung problems such as chronic cough, shortness of breath, pulmonary fibrosis (scarring and thickening of lung tissue), pleural effusion (accumulation of fluid between the membrane lining of the lung and chest cavity), and recurrent pneumonia.
- Decreased sex drive.
- Depression and thoughts of giving up or suicide.

Keep in mind that not all women susceptible to silicone-associated connective tissue disease will experience every symptom and that the degree of severity varies widely according to each individual's duration and extent of exposure, as well as her genetic makeup and immune system. These signs and symptoms also occur in patients without breast implants; however, the more indicators that are present in the absence of any obvious medical explanation make problems from silicone more likely.

As mentioned earlier, unfortunately there's no one blood test or other technique that can confirm the presence of silicone-induced autoimmune disease. Batteries of test results have varied widely from woman to woman. For example, there have been reports of patients with silicone-related symptoms who have cholesterol levels of over 480 (under 200 is ideal) and white blood cell counts of 33,000 per cubic millimeter of blood (normal range is 4,500 to 11,000), while others with the same symptoms have had normal test results. In fact, with the exception of uric acid crystals (gout) or bacteria growing in joint fluid, testing for rheumatic conditions rarely confirms a diagnosis; nor do test results determine treatment.

Although still inconclusive, the following results have been found to correlate with the disease in some implant recipients:

- Elevated sedimentation rate, a non-specific measure of inflammation in the body, based on the presence of certain proteins in the blood, has shown up in about 24 percent of patients.
- Elevated levels of antinuclear antibodies (ANA), which are antibodies that tend to react with components of cell nuclei. (ANA tests are positive in 30 percent of patients with silicone implants, but in only 1 percent to 2 percent of the general population.)

- Positive test for toxic porphyria, a disorder caused by overaccumulation in the body of coproporphyrin. *Porphyrins* are chemicals that play a key role in the manufacture of hemoglobin and other important body substances. Symptoms of porphyria may include extreme sensitivity to light, a rash, skin blistering, abdominal pain, and nervous system disturbances. (At the University of South Florida, a small number of women treated with implant-related problems have tested positive for this condition and their tests returned to normal after implant removal.)

I was a perfectly healthy, normal person, according to my medical tests . . . .

Doctors at her Health Maintenance Organization (HMO) didn't know what to make of Valerie's swollen glands, low-grade fever, chronic fatigue, diarrhea, hot flashes, pelvic pain, and symptoms of depression. She had a barium enema, sonogram, mammogram, blood tests, and urine tests, but nothing was revealed. There was blood in her stool, but tests showed no intestinal disease. She had severe pain near her gallbladder, but tests showed no problem with the organ. She had had implants since she was 18. "I was getting scared and frustrated, wondering why everybody else at work—women twenty and thirty years older than me—had so much more energy and felt OK," said Valerie. "All my tests always came out perfect. I was the only one out of all my friends and relatives having all these things going on. I just figured my body was weird and I had to live with it. I had to push myself because I didn't have the energy other people had. But the more I pushed, the more tired I got. It was a vicious cycle."

Later Valerie developed swelling in her face and eyelids. Her memory became so bad she thought she was developing Alzheimer's disease.

Finally, Valerie underwent more tests that confirmed a condition of toxic porphyria—a clear indication that something was poisoning her body. After having her implants out, she discovered that her mammogram results had not indicated that both her implants had in fact ruptured.

The Evidence Supporting a Relationship Between Silicone and Rheumatic Symptoms

If silicone and silica (silicon dioxide, the "parent" of silicone) were subjected to a trial, the jury would have much information to analyze before rendering a decision of guilty or not guilty regarding the endangering of women's health. The following points represent some of the most compelling evidence to date suggesting these materials as a perpetrator of autoimmune disorders.

1. Silica exposure is hazardous.

Silica has a well-documented record of damage to humans exposed to it on an ongoing basis. People in occupations such as sandblasting who inhale many silica particles may develop silicosis, a form of pulmonary fibrosis. This scarring and thickening of lung tissue usually results from inflammation and typically causes shortness of breath. In many cases, the condition is irreversible. When especially severe, it can lead to heart failure. Pulmonary fibrosis has been diagnosed in some USF breast implant patients.

2. Silica is an immunogen.

Silica (which is a sandlike material) is a proven immunogen, that is, a substance that stimulates the body's immune system to attack normal body tissue. The shell for both gel- and saline-filled implants is made of a polymer with a 30 percent silicon dioxide filler. The silica helps solidify the envelope, or implant jacket. Although it has not been proven to escape from the implant and enter the macrophages (the cells which ingest, kill, and digest foreign substances in the body), the gradual shedding of small particles from the outer shell of the implant makes immune-system exposure to a small but potentially critical amount of silica a real possibility requiring further study.

Since congregations of macrophages have been found on the surface of silicone implant jackets, it appears that these immune-system cells attack the jacket itself—whether or not silicone is leaking from it. In support of the shell-destruction/erosion hypothesis, Nir Kossovsky, a pathologist at University of California, Los Angeles (UCLA), has obtained compelling evidence using an electron microscopic X-ray technique on implants removed from patients.[15] Dr. Kossovsky, who presented his scientific findings to a congressional subcommittee, demonstrated how the body's macrophages attack the silicone shell of the breast implant. This process can be likened to gophers chewing into and through the implant's wall, chiseling off microscopic pieces of silicone, which then lodge in neighboring body tissue. Eventually, this cellular assault weakens the outer envelope to the point where it may rupture.

Silicone has been found in tissues peripheral to the breast even in the absence of implant rupture, which further implies that attacking macrophages can cause bits of the silicone envelope to break off. The immune process itself may also activate normal cells in the area. More research is required to determine the specifics of this process.

3. Animal and human studies show immune response.

Silicone oils were recognized as potential adjuvants in the 1960s by researchers. Adjuvants are substances that alter natural, "friendly" cells into activated cells capable of attacking the body.

Injections of silicone fluid under the skin in guinea pigs have produced severe granulomas (collections of macrophages). Granulomas have also been found in the breasts and livers of transsexual males who received silicone injections for breast enlargement. And epidemiological studies in Japan have reportedly shown substantial increases in specific rheumatic conditions in women who have received these injections.

Other toxicology research, conducted by implant manufacturers from the 1960s through the 1980s and provided to the FDA, indicates that various silicone compounds injected into mice, rabbits, monkeys, rats, and dogs can spread throughout the body. Macrophages containing silicone particles have been found in test animals' adrenal glands, lymph nodes, liver, kidney, spleen, pancreas, and ovaries. Results from Dow Corning's biosafety animal study reports have included findings of liver toxicity, stillbirths, fetal abnormalities, respiratory diseases, lesions, cancer, hemorrhages, and death. In mid-1982, for example, Dow initiated a project with an internal mammary gel formulation labeled Q7-2159A to address the issues of gel cohesivity and bleed, the results of which "showed the extreme sensitivity of the formulated gel to penetration and bleed." Further studies with this particular formulation, variously conducted over a decade, revealed "metastatic sarcomas," "enlarged lymph nodes," "pituitary adenomas," and "hair loss [that] may be associated with thyroid disorders." A subchronic toxicity study with formulation D5, contracted to the University of Mississippi Medical Center in 1989, found the gel to "induce [liver enlargement], with recovery after cessation of dosing," and it "resembled phenobarbital" in its ability to induce certain enzymatic activity.[16]

The potential of free silicone migration was also raised to company officials in at least one report submitted in 1976 by an outside testing laboratory. Injecting a series of gel formulations labeled TX 1228, TX 1229, and TX 1234, the researchers noted a "possibility that the test material may have migrated away from the implant sites."

When viewed under a microscope, tissue next to silicone implants has, in some women, shown an exceptionally high accumulation of scavenger cell-devouring macrophages. Unlike the finite healing of a particular wound, the assault of macrophages around the silicone implant does not stop, because the body continues to respond to the tiny, but potentially widespread, silicone particles.

In many women who receive silicone breast implants, the macrophages keep accumulating month after month, year after year. As more cells arrive, the scar tissue becomes increasingly thicker--often creating a series of hard, painful lumps or overall hardening of the breast, in addition to the likelihood of changes in the physical contour of the breast itself.

4. Silicone "bleeds" through, and sheds from, the envelope.

Numerous reports in the medical literature, as well as findings by manufacturers, have shown that a certain amount of silicone leaks, or "bleeds," through the outer casing of the implant jacket in every case, even when there is no rupture. This means that all women with silicone implants will experience some exposure to the gel.

Silicone particles may come off the outside of the envelope, perhaps creating potential hazard for women with saline-filled silicone envelope implants as well.

5. Silicone found in fibrous tissue around the implant.

Unpublished correlations between the amount of silicone in capsular tissue that surrounds an implant and the total amount of this tissue have been made by some researchers, but these findings have not yet been substantiated. The theory, however, is that silicone/silica appears directly related to the development of fibrosis, the overgrowth of scar or connective tissue around the prosthesis itself.

6. The body makes antibodies against silicone.

Studies conducted in the 1970s by John Paul Heggers of the University of Texas Medical Center at Galveston showed that the human immune system reacts to silicone in breast implants by making antibodies against it, according to a January 18, 1992, news report in the *New York Times*.[17] He found that these antibodies (which help macrophages and other immune-system components to destroy harmful invaders) attacked the silicone *as well as the body's own tissues* associated with it—a classic symptom of an autoimmune disorder. More such studies need to be conducted to confirm and isolate specific antibodies created by the body against silicone.

7. Epidemiologic studies show symptoms among breast implant recipients.

Michael Weisman, a rheumatologist at the University of California, San Diego, published a survey in a 1988 issue of the *Journal of Plastic and Reconstructive Surgery* of women who underwent silicone implant surgery for cosmetic purposes during a 12-year period. Of 125 women, 30 percent reported rheumatic complaints. None of the patients had rheumatoid arthritis or scleroderma, causing Weisman to believe it was a negative study. About 30 percent of the responding women (average age: 48) had musculoskeletal complaints. There was no control group for comparison.[18]

USF's Divisions of Plastic Surgery, Dermatology, and Rheumatology pursued the silicone-rheumatic disease connection further in 1988 with a survey of 370 women who had received silicone-gel breast implants and a control group who had undergone nonsilicone plastic surgery procedures. The women in the silicone group had had their implants for an average of five years, and their average age was 37. The average age of the control group was 46.

Even though the women in the silicone group averaged six years younger than the control group, they were discovered to be eight times more likely to suffer from tender lymph nodes under the arm (8 percent) than the control group (1 percent), as well as four times more likely to develop swollen lymph nodes under the arm (12 percent vs. 3 percent, respectively). Muscle pain, joint pain, joint swelling, and chronic fatigue were more common in the silicone patients, but these symptoms did not reach the 95 percent certainty level.

8. More symptoms occur near implant location.

In some women who have only one silicone implant due to unilateral mastectomy or breast asymmetry, symptoms of pain and inflammation tend to be more pronounced on the side of the body where the implant is located. Some of these women, as well as women known to have experienced a rupture in only one breast, have developed muscle pain and swelling in the arm on the affected side only. This asymmetrical reaction implies that a localized stimulation of the immune system occurs in the affected area.

9. Connective tissue disease in women with breast implants may differ from the naturally occurring disease.

Lupus: One of the first cases of silicone-associated connective tissue disease seen at USF was a woman treated for a condition similar to systemic lupus erythematosus (SLE) in 1987. This case was distinguished by a milky fluid with a high fat content in the membrane that lines the lungs and chest cavity, a condition known as chylous pleural effusion. We could find no similar reports of this specific problem occurring previously in natural SLE. Apparently, the woman's thoracic duct (a large duct of the lymphatic system located between the neck and the abdomen) had been inflamed and blocked by silicone granules and/or activated immune cells.

After she had her implants removed and was treated with cortisone, her symptoms resolved within six months. When the cortisone was stopped, her symptoms did not recur. Similar complete remissions have occurred in the natural disease, but are unusual. She continues to do well five years later.

Scleroderma: While this serious condition is extremely rare in the general population—approximately 50 cases per million people—a sclerodermalike illness has been documented in numerous women with silicone implants.

Steve Weiner, a Los Angeles–based rheumatologist, sent out a questionnaire to the Scleroderma Foundation and found 50 such women in the Los Angeles area alone.

Harry Spiera, a rheumatologist based in New York City, has reported that 4.4 percent of his scleroderma patients have implants—as opposed to only 0.3 percent of his rheumatoid arthritis patients. Although the percentages are low in both of these groups, what is significant is that he found over 14 times as many of his implant patients suffering from scleroderma as nonimplant patients.[19]

In the medical literature, about half the women with scleroderma have improved after implant removal, whereas remission of natural scleroderma without treatment occurs uncommonly.

Lung diseases: Studies of patients at USF show that some of those who have connective tissue disease also have lung disease. This suggests that silicone and possibly silica can make their way past regional lymph nodes into the right side of the heart and out to the lungs. This could result in lung inflammation and/or fibrosis.

Lucy Love and Fred Miller, at the FDA, reported an interesting clinical difference between naturally occurring dermatomyositis/polymyositis and the same disease in women with breast implants.[20] The implant patients were found to have a higher prevalence of pulmonary fibrosis than nonimplant patients (about 50 percent versus 20 percent). Although this observation is preliminary since it is based on fewer than 20 women with implants who have the disease, it nonetheless suggests that implants are playing a role in this illness.

Sjögren's Syndrome: Additionally, Bruce Freundlich, a rheumatologist from the University of Pennsylvania, reported at the American College of Rheumatology meeting in October 1992 that women with breast implants exhibited the immune-mediated symptoms of dry eyes and dry mouth.[21]

10. Chronic fatigue and swollen lymph nodes have been observed.

Many women with silicone disease suffer from chronic fatigue. Based on the USF 1988 questionnaire, 15 percent of the silicone group reported having chronic fatigue compared with only 11 percent in the control group without implants. Statistically, this is suggestive (more likely than not) but not definitive (that is, below 95 percent certain).

Also, clinical observation of lymph node swelling is more dramatic in silicone-related lupus and other connective tissue diseases than in nonsilicone versions of these diseases. Through a method not yet understood, silicone particles can enter the lymphatic system (a network of glands and fluid-carrying ducts) and become lodged in lymph nodes under the arm, in the neck, and in the groin. The silicone, combined with various immune-system cells, can then travel via the lymphatic system to stimulate a dangerous cycle of immune and lymphatic system "excitation," one that builds and builds. Should this occur, some women experience swollen and painful lymph nodes in their breasts, necks, underarms, and groin. This diverse swelling indicates that the immune system has been stimulated throughout the body, not just at the site of the implant.

As various immune cells migrate into the lymphatic channels, they soon enter the lymph nodes. In a complex process, they interact with other immune cells, particularly T-cell lymphocytes (which cause or facilitate tissue damage), causing the lymph nodes to enlarge and become repositories of "angry" immune cells. Views through a microscope reveal a condition called reactive hyperplasia, an overgrowth of the lymph node resulting from reactions to environmental factors—including silicone.

Scientists agree that microscopic quantities of silicone reach the lymph nodes along with immune cells. But there is disagreement over what happens to this substance once it settles in the nodes. Ultimately, silicone particles may be able to travel throughout the entire body. This may occur via the following process:

1. Lymph fluid goes into the chest in a tubelike collecting system called the thoracic duct.

2. This fluid, and possibly the silicone particles themselves, goes into the right side of the heart and into the lungs via the thoracic duct.

3. Once it flows past the lungs, the left side of the heart pumps the lymph and silicone particles out to the rest of the body. If this occurs, silicone will enter the bloodstream and may possibly trigger a bodywide immune-system response.

11. Implant removal results in improvement.

Of the first 50 women with silicone disease tracked at USF, 33 decided to have their prostheses removed. The result: *70 percent of these women felt better within two years*, with improvement occurring on average between 6 and 18 months following explantation. And while 30 percent did not show improvement, at least their symptoms stopped getting worse in all but one case. In these and hundreds of other patients treated and monitored at our Division of Rheumatology, the symptoms of women who have removed the implants have generally, although not uniformly, improved or resolved. (These observations, reported in October 1992 by *USA Today*, have been confirmed by William Shaw, Professor and Chief of Plastic Surgery at UCLA Medical Center, who also described improvement of systemic symptoms in 70 percent of 150 women who removed their implants.)

We must emphasize that the degree of improvement a patient will experience depends on how much silicone has leaked into her body, the duration of her exposure, and the susceptibility of her immune system. Thus, improvement can never be guaranteed.

Some doctors have claimed that alleviation of symptoms following explantation may be due to certain steroids produced by the body in response to the surgery itself. If that were true, postoperative improvements would be short-lived. In fact, many women experience permanent improvement after their implants are removed—even permanent cessation of their symptoms in some cases. (Note: Symptoms are often reported to worsen during the first few weeks after implant removal. This is not a cause for concern; it may be due to the freeing of more silicone by the surgical procedure, and is almost always temporary. Additionally, the benefit of emotional relief—the placebo effect—would be noted immediately.)

12. Implants may increase the risk of neurological disease.

Bernard M. Patten, a neurologist at Baylor College of Medicine in Houston, has found an association between silicone breast implants and serious autoimmune conditions as well as neurological dysfunction. In an August 27, 1992, abstract for a platform presentation to the American Neurological Association, he described several young women with amyotrophic lateral sclerosis (ALS), known as Lou Gehrig's disease and whose typical victims are older men, and many others who showed signs of sensory-motor neuropathy and other symptoms.[22] The average time of disease onset, Patten reported, was about seven years from implantation. In addition, some of these women had peripheral nerve disease, a condition not seen in the natural form of ALS.

Dr. Patten, in the same abstract submission, also reported on patients with implants who had an unusual form of multiple sclerosis (MS). These patients demonstrated a combination of typical MS symptoms along with the unexpected manifestation of joint pain and swelling. This highly unusual combination could mean that implants had been a factor in triggering a silicone-specific version of the condition. Symptoms were found to improve in some patients following implant removal. The neurologist's conclusion was that "silicone may provoke damage to nerve and muscle, probably indirectly promoting autoimmunity." In the research submitted for publication, he strongly recommends a "reappraisal of the risk-benefit ratio for [silicone breast implant] surgery."

13. Patients exhibit immune response to other silicone implants.

Problems from silicone are not limited to breast implants. USF rheumatologists observed a woman with severe osteoarthritis (wear and tear, degenerative, old-age arthritis) at the base of her thumb. She had had a solid silicone spacer placed in the joint. Over many months, the patient developed warmth and tenderness over the spacer, swollen lymph nodes in the area, and chronic fatigue. Upon removal of the silicone device, these problems resolved and no evidence of infection could be found. Other surgeons have reported unique radiographic lesions (holes in the wrist bones) in the carpal bones in patients with silicone devices implanted in their hands.

Another study showed that patients on kidney dialysis whose blood was pumped through silicone tubing contracted liver disease at an unusually high rate, according to a news report in *New York Times*.[23] Autopsies revealed a large number of silicone particles in the livers of these patients. When nonsilicone tubing was substituted, the incidence of liver disease dropped dramatically. Other problems have been noted to occur following cardiac bypass surgery, when silicone was used as an antifoam agent in devices that oxygenate the blood. Tiny particles of silicone escaped from the devices and blocked capillaries in these patients, causing tissue damage. On a positive note, however, silicone has been used with fewer reports of problems in other devices, including indwelling catheters, cardiac pacemakers, and artificial heart valves. Again, more research is required.

Foam Implants Pose Cancer Risk

Cigarette smoke, asbestos, radium, cyclamates, chromium, nickel, hardwood dusts—these are just a few of the many substances that at one time were thought harmless and have turned out to be contributors to cancer development. Today, these materials are known to take from 14 to 40 years to trigger cancer in humans. Polyurethane foam–covered implants may also join this lineup in the future.

Foam-coated implants were originally designed to help prevent the natural scar tissue around implants from developing into capsular contracture. Studies later showed that the outer layer of foam could break down in the body. A by-product of this breakdown is 2-toluene diamine (TDA), a substance that has been banned in hair dyes and other products because it causes liver cancer in animals.[24]

The late William J. Pangman, a prominent plastic surgeon who developed the foam used as a filler and coating for these implants, claimed that the foam shouldn't break down in the human body. Yet no one seems to have a record of exactly what kind of foam he used. (See chapter 4 for a full discussion.) Today, an estimated 10 percent of women who have silicone-gel implants have foam-coated prostheses. They were taken off the market in February 1991.

Additionally, while there is no *documented* association between silicone and cancer, studies to date have been inadequate. (The FDA has advised women with these implants, however, not to have them removed because the risk of cancer, if any, is presently deemed to be low.) Research is ongoing.

Women with No Symptoms: Is There a Need to Worry?

Many women have suffered no setbacks years after receiving silicone-gel implants. For others, symptoms began mere months after implantation. Unfortunately, there's no way of predicting when or if symptoms will occur in any woman.

All assumptions about silicone disease are based on the limited evidence accumulated to date. The conditions of perhaps hundreds of thousands of women with implants have yet to be assessed. Some of those who feel healthy now may in the past have had temporary silicone-related symptoms, but breast capsule formation may have acted to reduce the flow of silicone particles from the implant, or perhaps in some individuals the immune system adjusted to the silicone and, possibly, silica exposure as well.

What Medical Studies Are Needed?

Many factors must be explored in greater depth to fill in the gaps of the silicone disease puzzle. While many doctors believe that there is at least the possibility of a connection, more definitive proof of a cause-effect relationship is needed to satisfy most practitioners in the medical establishment.

Just as some smokers puff away into old age while others die of lung cancer in their forties, women's susceptibility to silicone may also vary widely. This is precisely why it is vital to gather data on many more women than the small groups of patients investigated by individual physicians thus far. Only well-designed studies, involving thousands of women, will reveal the degree to which silicone implants are likely to trigger autoimmune diseases. These studies may yield information for people with other types of silicone implants as well.

In addition, a national implant and explant registry needs to be established by the FDA. This registry would enable the FDA to be notified about any breast implant that is removed and the reasons for removal. All removed specimens could then be processed at an *independent* centralized laboratory for analysis, thereby overcoming the biases of individual surgeons or physicians.

Also, Medic Alert, in Turlock, California, has begun a program to enroll women with breast implants and, for a small fee, to provide them and their physicians with the latest information.

Several key topics regarding silicone disease require more investigation:

1. Patient Predisposition

Some women may have immune systems that are especially vulnerable to silicone exposure and are easily triggered into an autoimmune response. Screening procedures need to be developed to help doctors identify these women and to evaluate the roles played by a previously weakened immune system; hormonal factors; smoking and use of alcohol and other drugs; history of disease or trauma; interactions between silicone and other biological substances; environmental factors; types of physical activity; ethnic background; and other complex factors in the development of silicone-related disease.

2. Genetic Markers for Silicone Sensitivity

Can silicone sensitivity be inherited? Do some women have genes that make them more likely to reject silicone in their bodies? Research efforts such as the Human Genome Project may one day lead us toward recognition of genetic predeterminants of everything from life span to cancer risk. People with similar rheumatic conditions have been shown to have certain genetic markers, so perhaps there are "fingerprints" for susceptibility to silicone disease as well—or conversely, a set of genes that make a person *immune* from the disease. For example, the FDA's Fred Miller, a rheumatologist, found a genetic marker (HLA DQA10102) in women who have dermatomyositis/polymyositis and breast implants that is much more common than it is in women without implants who have these diseases. And at USF, we observed a set of identical twins with implants who both presented the same symptoms in a similar time frame. This common course implies a genetic component toward predisposition, which, if confirmed, could make it possible for women one day to be tested for susceptibility. Women who have no symptoms but who test positive could have their implants taken out before the disease launches its first offensive. Similarly, women with the genetic predisposition could avoid placing the implants in the first place.

3. Silicone Gel as Adjuvant

Can silicone serve as an *adjuvant* (or immune enhancer) that results in the formation of new substances in the body that get wrongly defined as enemies by the immune system? Maybe. Most previous studies asserting that silicone could have this function are based on direct injections of silicone, however, which typically include silicone mixed with other substances.

Another concern that must be investigated is whether the autoimmune response activated by silicone is self-perpetuating. If this occurs, removal of silicone from the body will not be enough to stop the disease from progressing. This may occur in some patients and not others, and individuals may also have different self-perpetuating "trigger" thresholds.

4. How Silicone Spreads in the Body

Some women with implants which rupture show no symptoms beyond the chest area; others may end up with silicone traveling throughout the body, with traces of it in the liver, ovaries, and other organs, as well as joints and muscles. Research needs to determine all the aspects of anatomy, body chemistry, and other factors that expedite migration of silicone particles within the body, as well as to teach us the mechanisms that allow silicone to travel through the lymphatic system.

More comprehensive urinalyses and studies at the molecular level may also help determine whether tiny particles of silicone can find their way into the bloodstream. If they can, this news could be especially disturbing, suggesting that silicone can very easily find its way to the heart and other internal organs. It is reassuring, however, that heart, kidney, and liver failure have not been observed in women seen at USF.

5. Breast Implant as Infection "Ally"

One theory proposes that leaked silicone gel or the envelope itself could provide a hiding place for infectious agents, particularly bacteria or fungi within the body. If the immune system cannot detect these "invisible" infections, it cannot attack them; the hidden invaders can then multiply and reach critical levels that overwhelm the immune system once they spread throughout the body. Experiments with silicone and infectious agents in the laboratory are needed to assess this hypothesis. More careful and precise methods of study of the removed breast capsule could help answer these questions.

6. Silicone as Carcinogen

So far, only animal studies have confirmed a causal link between silicone exposure and cancer, according to data obtained from the FDA and Dow and reported by The Public Citizen Health Research Group, a nonprofit consumer group.[25] While some animal studies have reportedly shown a significant increase in cancer risk in areas of the body other than the breast among implant recipients, other studies have been inconclusive.[26] Additional studies must be performed to confirm or refute this connection. Cancer is often the result of long-term exposure to an activating substance, and many women have had implants for only a few years—so it is difficult at this time to know the real risks. Women with implants need to be monitored for many years to see if their cancer rates are higher than those for the general population. A reassuring Canadian study was recently published in the *New England Journal of Medicine*, however.[27]

7. Effects of Implantation

Implants that are nicked during surgery increase the risk of leakage and make the prosthesis especially prone to rupture. What isn't known is how likely it is for such damage to occur during implantation. Data are also lacking on whether the implantation procedure and resultant structural change due to surgery can cause late-developing musculoskeletal pains due to direct disruption of tissue planes, ligaments, or nerves. Is there a difference depending upon whether the implants are placed on top of or behind the chest muscles? Also, further exploration is needed to determine whether implants play a role in infection. (The skin over the breasts of women who receive implants following mastectomy is sometimes incapable of holding implants in place, due to the trauma of chemotherapy, radiation, and previous surgery.)

8. New Body Configuration

As a result of anatomical accommodation of implants by the body, pains in the chest wall, shoulders, and neck may be due to changes in posture, weight, and body biomechanics. This hypothesis is unlikely, but needs to be explored more fully by comparing implant recipients with other women whose body configurations have been changed in similar ways.

9. Rate of Shell Breakdown

While small amounts of silicone "bleed" through the silicone rubber casing, the life span of these casings within the body remains unknown, though implants were never intended to be once-in-a-lifetime prostheses. The rate at which shells break down, how much silicone bleeds through them, and what kind of trauma can cause rupture— these factors need to be better studied.

Artificial joint implants made of silicone that were placed in the 1960s are now reaching a point when material fatigue predisposes them to fracture. And while today's new breast implants can reportedly withstand tremendous pressure per square inch, what happens over time with loss of silicone from the envelope? And how vulnerable are implants to puncture by surgical instruments, needles, and broken ribs? Characteristics that have value in predicting future performance—such as tensile strength and fatigue resistance—need to be precisely determined by hundreds of trials.

10. What Happens to Gel in Body Tissues?

This issue opens a huge number of unanswered questions. Does the chemical composition of the gel change after it leaks into the body? Is silicone metabolized in the tissues? How can silicone-induced connective tissue disease be distinguished from "standard" connective tissue disease on a chemical basis? Is there a way to measure antibodies associated with silicone exposure? While some evidence shows silicone may cause changes in molecular structure, much research is still needed to answer all of these questions. In addition, it needs to be determined whether certain organs are more sensitive than others to silicone.

11. Silicone as a Threat to the Fetus and Newborn

Also still to be determined is whether silicone that escapes from an implant can penetrate the placental barrier and adversely affect an unborn child. Additionally, we need to explore whether leaking silicone can end up in breast milk (women with implants are not recommended to breast-feed), and how the breast-feeding infant may be affected by its consumption. Further, it has been theorized that the implantation procedure itself may restrict some blood supply to the milk-producing system, or apply pressure to milk-collecting sacs, not allowing them to expand and thereby reducing milk flow or supply.

12. Emotional Disorders and Silicone Disease

Are rheumatic disorders from silicone exposure playing a role in such emotional problems as depression, anxiety/panic, even chronic fatigue syndrome? Definitive criteria for determining a causal link need to be established. Many case studies make it clear that patients become depressed, enraged, even suicidal, over their illness. But is silicone itself a depressant, or are these women's emotional disorders purely a reaction to their symptoms?

13. Silicone and Sexuality

Numerous women have reported a drastic fall in libido, if not a total loss of sex drive, during the downward course of their silicone-related illness. Is this the result of their feeling poorly all the time, or their feeling self-hate over their physical appearance? Or does silicone exposure have a specific and deleterious effect on the sex drive itself? The experiences of many more women will have to be documented to clarify this issue.

"You go from flat-chested to something. And it's like, oh, wow, I really look good! But after a woman gets sick and has her implants out, it's like ending up with a radical mastectomy. Then they are left worse than before," Cecilia commented, having gone through this experience herself. "Women don't want to talk about it because they can't deal with this issue."

Patients who have gone through an involved explantation have described how in order to gain support emotionally they get together with other women in the same position, pull their shirts off, and compare. Joyce remarked, "It's scary . . . scary what we look like. A lot take showers in the dark. They do not undress in front of their husbands, or allow themselves to be seen nude. You can imagine what this does to a marriage. Women are humiliated.

"It's devastating enough for a woman either not to have breasts or lose them the first time," Joyce continued. "But when you have to go back and lose them for a second time, it's really more than what a normal person can bear."

"I still have a chest, if you want to call it that," Cecilia added. "My last mammogram showed 36 different silicone granulomas, and one breast is larger than the other. I'm looking at more surgery to get the silicone out, but it really can't be retrieved. I'm past embarrassed. I could pull off my shirt on TV and it wouldn't faze me. I don't care anymore," she lamented.

"Women have to realize that they are the same person they were before they lost their breasts," Joyce explained. "It's still me. My husband, well, he has to love me for what I am on the inside, not what I look like on the outside. If that's the only thing a man cares about, it's not worth trying to stay in the marriage to begin with."

14. Silicone Gel versus Saline Gel Implants

Although saline (salt water) is harmless to the body if it leaks, it should be noted that saline-filled implants are encased in a silicone rubber envelope that may shed silicone particles into the body. Many women who have had silicone-gel implants removed only to have them replaced with saline-filled implants may not be in the position of safety they assume. More studies comparing the pros and cons of the two types of implants are presently required by the FDA and are now underway.

It's the saline, too . . . .

Margo worked as an office manager for a physician, running three ob/gyn offices. With saline implants following reconstruction from fibrocystic disease, she began to get tired just a few months after getting the prostheses. Her problems with saline implants were as bad as any woman with silicone gel–induced illness.

"I was just tired," she said. "Then I kept getting the same flu and weird rashes. I had horrid chest pains as time went on and terrible pain in my muscles. I was diagnosed as having one virus or flu after another. I even wondered if I had contracted AIDS, because I had had every viral study you could imagine done. I was at my wits' end." Margo was finally diagnosed as having lupus and silicone-associated connective tissue disease in 1989 at the USF Department of Rheumatology.

She reported, "People are aware of the dangers of silicone implants, but we've got sick women with saline implants, too. I just don't think there's a safe implant on the market."

15. Treatment

At this time the only treatment for silicone-induced disease is to rid the body of all silicone, by removing the implants and fibrous tissue around them. We need to seek vigorously more effective ways to detoxify the entire body of silicone particles, and to develop drug treatments targeted specifically to conditions caused by silicone. Identification of antibodies against silicone produced by the body would greatly expedite this research. Symptomatic relief for some patients has been found in aspirin and the aspirinlike medications called nonsteroidal anti-inflammatory drugs like Motrin, Naproxen, Indocin, Feldene, and others. In severe circumstances, cortisone, Plaquenil, and other immunosuppressive approaches could be used.

Here's our idea of a perfect study. All women who have implants should be monitored by a rheumatologist once a year for 20 years after implantation. For each implant recipient monitored, another woman of similar age and health who has no implants should be monitored at the same intervals. The prevalence of back pain, neck pain, fibromyalgia, swollen lymph nodes, swollen joints, chronic fatigue, and other autoimmune functions would be checked in both groups.

Such a study would yield mountains of conclusive data about the course of silicone disease and its true significance in women with implants. Unfortunately, it would demand a lot of effort and cost a fortune.

And who should pay for it? Of all the questions asked so far about silicone disease, this may be the toughest to answer. Although USF recently received $15,000 from the St. Petersburg Medical Clinic to pursue the connection between silicone and disease, it is only a drop in the bucket considering what is needed to generate definitive results.

I think it's a crime they're getting away with this . . . .

When several women told their plastic surgeons about their silicone-related problems, the doctors just made jokes about them; one told his patient she had "Connie Chung disease," referring to the TV broadcast in December 1990 that catapulted silicone disease onto the national agenda. But this surgeon is not making jokes anymore: several of his implant patients are now suing him.

After Ms. Chung's segment, Sally Jesse Raphael and many other talk-show hosts rushed to cover silicone implants. Most of these segments have been human interest stories, however; there has been insufficient time and focus devoted to hard-core facts and medical science. And many "news bites," while serving to bring the silicone implant issue under scrutiny, have also served to tease or frighten viewers with incomplete or mistaken information.

Soon after the Chung special, testimony before Congress on silicone disease by several experts, including Frank Vasey, garnered surprisingly little interest from reporters, none of whom sought further comments. However, Dr. Vasey's five minutes of testimony ended up on CNN, broadcast across the country, and women were watching; the phone at the USF Department of Rheumatology has been ringing with cries for help from implant victims ever since. New patients must now wait over a year to see him.

Implants in the Courtroom

Silicone-gel implants are not just a health problem—they've become a major legal problem as well. Settlements in the multimillion-dollar range have been awarded to some women who have taken on implant manufacturers in the courtroom and won. Recently, however, manufacturers have won two cases in Colorado. Countless others are now suing their surgeons for malpractice.

Yet all the attention given to these lawsuits may backfire; it could trigger greed in some women who do not really suffer from silicone disease but who pack the courts with sophisticated legal wrangling. Thousands of women are presently waiting their turn to testify about their implants. The end result of this could be a backlash that works against women who really deserve significant compensation for their silicone-induced suffering. Sadly, we live today in a highly litigious world. The law, originally developed to defend the innocent, has evolved culturally into a powerful assault vehicle. A flood of legal battles are thus likely in which even the winners will lose, given the energy, expense, and emotional trauma involved in extracting a victory.

Further, several cases have been consolidated for discovery (i.e., depositions and expert testimony) under Judge Pointer in the northern district of Alabama. Negotiations for a settlement are ongoing.

Disability Claims

Thousands of women are partially or completely disabled as a result of silicone disease. Since the medical establishment has not yet officially recognized the "validity" of this illness, the social security administration and the medical insurance companies have denied claim after claim for desperately needed medical benefits. There have even been reports of insurance companies canceling the policies of women following noncovered explantation, with other carriers changing policy wording to avoid future liability.

It has been hypothesized that the social security system may nevertheless soon have to change its stance regarding the denial of silicone disease claims, due to the steadily growing number of illnesses being reported. And with the SSI funding crisis, a failing disability program is a horrifying prospect, especially in light of the denials by private health insurance carriers. Where will it leave these women and their families, unable to pay their health care bills, unable to work, draining family savings to make ends meet?

In a worst-case scenario, should it turn out years from now that 10 percent of all implant recipients do become sick, that represents a staggering 100,000 or more women who risk disability. Women with silicone disease have a legitimate medical disability and cannot work. Many feel as though they've been "run over by a truck" day after day. Pressure needs to be put on the government, the insurance companies, and the health care profession to acknowledge these issues and to address them fairly.

The Double Standard of Medical Research

The long reign of silicone implants as "completely safe" fits right into the sad tradition in the United States of taking women's health less seriously than men's. This is hardly the first time that women have been shortchanged by the medical establishment.

Case in point: Research into heart disease in this country has often excluded women entirely. Adding insult to injury, research findings have often been discussed as if they applied to both sexes. For example, numerous long-term studies showing that regular doses of aspirin can help prevent heart attack or stroke recurrence were done entirely with men. We know very little about risk factors that may affect women selectively.

Anecdotal evidence also suggests that women are less likely to be given diagnostic workups and treatment by medical professionals with as much care as men would receive. When doctors can find no obvious physical reason for a woman's complaint, they often consider it emotional in origin. Many women treated in this fashion, certainly those with silicone disease, have suffered needlessly, often believing that their problems were psychosomatic.

Thalidomide, DES, the Dalkon Shield—it seems that many of medical history's worst blunders have made women their chief victims. Just a coincidence? Although it's beyond the scope of this book to dig deeply into this shameful issue, we can only hope that the silicone disaster will give us enough perspective to prevent a recurrence. In our opinion what has happened to women with implants in this country is a form of downright abuse.

If I didn't get them out, I'm convinced I would have died . . . .

When Helen told her plastic surgeon about the problems she and other women with implants were having, he told her that they were all probably just having a bad case of premenstrual syndrome (PMS). Although she had an impulse to strangle him, she partly trusted him. The reverence toward doctors as gods had long been instilled in her.

She saw about 20 other doctors over a three-year period, during which she had problems ranging from severe digestive difficulties and numbing fatigue to memory lapses and vaginal infections that wouldn't clear up. She told those doctors all about the implants, but not one paid any attention. An endocrinologist took her aside and told her to repeat ten times after him, "It is not my implants." "I felt like no one wanted to help me," she said.

More than a year after her implants were removed, Helen feels better. She is convinced that she would not be alive if she had kept them in.

This chapter has dealt with the medical side of silicone disease. Next, we'll look at the immune system.

Chapter 3

How Silicone Affects the Body's Immune System

He tugged and tugged and pulled to get them out. At times he was lifting me off the table . . . .

Ellen received her implants just after graduating from college. Her health rapidly deteriorated to the point where she was having 20 bowel movements a day. Doctors prescribed a series of antibiotics and gave her Vitamin B shots for exhaustion, but nothing helped. Repeated CAT scans kept revealing new problems: an enlarged liver, a tumor on her kidney, a swollen adrenal gland. "I thought I had cancer and they weren't telling me," she said.

While windsurfing one day, Ellen felt something pull across the inside of her chest. From that moment on, she suffered from severe inflammation in her rib cage, as well as pains in her chest, muscles, and joints. Her plastic surgeon told her to "go home and take aspirin." She felt as if she was burning up and had to sleep with ice packs. She eventually lost her job as well as her social life. All she could do was stay home and rest. Her memory was also becoming unreliable; she was increasingly afraid to drive because she would often get lost—even when driving to places she had gone to hundreds of times before.

Finally, Ellen went to see a rheumatologist, who suggested that she have her implants removed. She cried for two days before the surgery, but was convinced that it was the right decision.

During the explantation, the surgeon cut through the original incisions to retrieve Ellen's implants, which had been inserted submuscularly. "He had to cut through all that muscle to get them out," she said. "And they didn't pop right out. It was a tug-of-war game. He tugged and tugged and pulled to get them out. At times, he was lifting me off the table. I could feel my skin burning. I could feel him cutting. I could smell it, hear it sizzling, and I told him I could feel that. He didn't . . . he didn't acknowledge it.

"At that point, after he got one implant, I told him I wanted to keep them, please do not throw them away, I wanted to have them analyzed. Again, he didn't acknowledge that I was talking to him. I started shaking. I pulled my legs up a little bit, and the only thing he said to me during the whole procedure was to put my legs down. I felt I was going into shock. My legs felt as though I was just going to bounce off the table.

"There was a nurse in the room, but she had told me before the procedure—this was so weird—that she hadn't been nursing for three years. She had been called in that week because the regular nurse was on vacation. So during the middle of the procedure, the surgeon started yelling for his office manager to put the phones on night service and to come back there, it was going to take three people to do this. I started shaking and trembling. It was very traumatic."

After the operation, the surgeon refused to release Ellen's implants to her. She had to hire an attorney to get her implants returned from the manufacturer. But she never knew for sure whether they were really hers.

A year after explantation, Ellen feels a lot better but still fatigues easily. "It just comes down to this point. Do you want to live or do you want larger breasts?"

Ellen's body, like the bodies of all women with silicone-associated connective tissue disease, had developed a powerful and worsening immune-system response to silicone. Her explantation experience was terrifying, but few are that traumatizing. As horrific as it was for her, she did not regret it—given that recovery from her silicone disease symptoms began shortly following the surgery.

In this chapter, we will examine the body's intricate immune system in order to understand precisely how silicone acts to trigger violent rheumatic and autoimmune illnesses in susceptible individuals. We'll also take a closer look at rheumatic diseases: what they are and how they can affect us. The more patients and physicians understand the connection between silicone disease and the immune system, the closer we will come to rapid medical diagnosis, treatment, and perhaps even prevention.

The Immune-System Militia

Imagine an army so well equipped and trained it could obliterate virtually every enemy force, an army so on guard that even a single infiltrator would be detected and destroyed almost immediately, before damage could be done.

This description is not a fantasy. Rather, it is an apt summary of the body's immune system—our personal armed forces on a continuous search-and-destroy mission, capable of protecting our bodies against invisible invaders 24 hours a day throughout our lives.

Our miraculous immune system, though exceptionally tough, is not invincible. Sometimes it can be overcome, as in a losing battle with cancer; other times it can be tricked into turning upon itself, due to some inherent defect or a foreign material—such as silicone. Such immune-system mutiny, to be discussed at length in this chapter, results from the body's inability to differentiate healthy body cells from dangerous invader cells and therefore blindly attacking everything in sight. In effect, the body begins to destroy its own immune system via "friendly fire." When this occurs (the definition of autoimmune disease), the result is the initiation of a devastating cellular civil war.

How the Body's Immune System Protects Us

Our immune system, 1 trillion white blood cells strong, defends and protects us against all invasions of bacteria, debris, and other disease-producing substances that threaten our health. Effective functioning of this system requires adequate supplies of the following "weapons":

- *Neutrophils*, which attack bacteria, make up about 60 percent of the white blood cells circulating in our bloodstream.

- *Lymphocytes* make up an additional 30 percent of our white blood cells, which are composed of B cells and two types of T cells:

  B cells act as a kind of biological arms factory, producing invader-fighting antibodies.

  Helper T cells, the "generals" of the immune-system army, facilitate tissue damage by identifying invading enemies and stimulating production of other infection-fighting cells.

  Killer T cells, recruited and activated by Helper T cells, serve to kill body cells that have been invaded by foreign organisms.

- *Monocytes*, which transform white blood cells into larger, attack-oriented elements called *macrophages* when they leave the blood and enter the tissues, are cells that ingest, kill, and digest foreign substances throughout our bodies.

- *Antibodies* are protein substances that the body creates to enable macrophages, neutrophils, and T cells to zero in on and destroy specific harmful bacteria and viral invaders.

Of these four basic components, the macrophages are the true front-line defenders of the immune-system army. They work tirelessly in our tissues to find and dispose of toxins, surround and neutralize illness-producing bacteria, and secrete hormonelike substances that attract and spark other immune-system helper T cell allies into action. Macrophages attack foreign substances like an amoeba (a one-celled protozoan) by encircling, consuming, and neutralizing them.

Rounding out our immune-system arsenal are antibodies, which circulate in both the bloodstream and the lymphatic system (the network of glands and fluid-carrying channels and ducts). Antibodies act to "tie up" and "tag" foreign invaders so they can be captured and eliminated by other members of our cellular militia.

When all immune-system components are working properly, the body conducts a battle against an invader in four basic stages:

1. Macrophages spot invaders and rapidly consume some of them. They then signal, and help activate, other members of the immune system into action.

2. The immune system forces multiply: helper T cells get involved, as do killer T cells and B cells. Antibodies are eventually stimulated as the number of B cells and helper T cells increases.

3. Killer T cells begin to destroy invaders by chemically puncturing their membranes, enabling antibodies to bind to the surface of the invaders in order to stop the "bad guys" from attacking other cells. They also destroy the foreign offenders directly. In this way, the offending invasion is conquered.

4. After the offensive is contained, a third type of T cells, called suppressor T cells, enters the scene. These T cells serve to slow and finally stop the overall immune system response, returning everything to a normal, "prewar," vigilant status.

Healthy people have two types of immunity provided by antibodies:

1. Natural (nonspecific) Immunity

This protection is present in the body at birth and requires no prior exposure to bacteria or toxins to be stimulated into action. Natural antibodies patrol the body on the lookout for unwanted, dangerous intruders. Heredity also plays an important role in the strength and effectiveness of natural immunity, varying from individual to individual and even among siblings in the same family.

2. Acquired (specific) Immunity

This protection occurs when the body learns to recognize and neutralize a substance that is not its own. The learning process may occur naturally—for example, by exposure to a substance in the environment or through immunization. Immunization is the introduction of either killed or weakened bacteria or viral substances into the body to stimulate production of protective antibodies against a specific disease. After our antibodies easily defeat the intentionally introduced, weakened enemy, they remain in circulation, prepared to attack and rapidly destroy any larger, stronger force of the given invader, should it ever again enter our system.

Distinguishing the Good from the Bad

The ability of the immune system to distinguish dangerous invaders from the body's own healthy cells is critical to the maintenance of our well-being. Since foreign substances can become interspersed throughout healthy tissue, accurate targeting of the immune system against invaders is essential; even a near miss by well-intentioned, attacking antibodies can destroy useful cells. Hence, the body must produce a wide range of different antibodies to strike against specific bacteria (just as a "smart bomb" zeros in on a specific target and hits it). These include both natural and acquired antibodies.

Shifting our analogy a bit, antibodies act as bloodhounds that have been given a piece of a criminal's clothing to sniff. Once they know the scent of their prey, they track the target relentlessly, ignoring all else during their pursuit. Providing that the immune system is functioning properly, innocent bystanders—that is, healthy adjacent cells—do not get hurt. Problems occur, however, when levels of bacteria or toxic substances reach a critical point at which the immune system gets overwhelmed, as when a foreign material, such as silicone, gets into the body. As described in the previous chapters, derailing the immune system, for any reason, can lead to unpredictable and highly destructive consequences.

Why Silicone Triggers the Immune System

In case studies presented throughout this book, each woman has been shown to suffer from a chronic systemic ailment that would not get better. Time and again doctors could detect no reasons for these problems: one drug after another failed to work, even though the medication's effectiveness was well documented. In each case, silicone had "confused" the patient's immune system to the point where it began fighting the body itself. The body no longer recognized who was an enemy or an ally and attacked both.

This type of immune-system attack may be local—affecting a specific area of the body—or systemic, meaning the entire body is affected. There are three basic reasons why the immune system can be triggered into action by a silicone implant:

1. Silicone escapes from the implant into surrounding body tissue.

As discussed, implants themselves bleed silicone through their outer silicone jackets even in the absence of overt rupture. The silicone envelope is also recognized as an invader by the immune system following implantation. As a result, cells are quickly directed to the invasion site to initiate a steady and ever-increasing attack upon the enemy (the implant's foreign outer shell). The body's macrophages zero in on the implant's envelope and encase it, a process (described in chapter 2) believed to lead to the slow destruction of the shell itself. This process of shell erosion, in turn, leads to further shedding of silicone molecules into the tissues surrounding the implant, whipping up the immune system still more. (Such an erosion effect has been similarly noted in patients with saline implants, which also have silicone outer shells.) Should destruction of the shell reach a point at which a hole is created by the macrophage attacks, silicone gel can leak steadily into the body. This situation also leaves open the increased possibility of outright rupture.

2. Silicone particles migrate throughout the lymphatic system.

Through a method not yet understood, silicone particles can enter the lymphatic system and become lodged in lymph nodes under the arm, in the neck, and in the groin. Then the silicone can combine with immune-system cells and travel via the lymphatic system to regional lymph nodes, where their presence stimulates more lymphocytes to respond to the foreign material. Once again, a cycle of immune and lymphatic system excitation begins, one that builds and builds. Some women experience swollen and painful lymph nodes in the breasts, neck, underarms, and groin. This diverse swelling indicates that the immune system has been stimulated at a distance from the implant. Serious rheumatic illnesses can result.

3. Macrophages conglomerate around silicone.

When viewed under a microscope, tissue next to silicone implants has, in some women, shown an exceptionally high accumulation of scavenger cell-devouring macrophages. In mass groupings, macrophages often join together to form a unified fighting force. The unity of action among these cells is often enhanced further by release of hormonelike substances, known as interleukins, that improve communication and cooperation among the cells. This conglomeration of macrophages causes a thickening of tissue around the implant that is similar to the process of wound healing; a scar forms, with the scar tissue typically thicker and denser than normal tissue.

However, unlike the finite healing of a particular wound, the assault of macrophages around the silicone implant does not stop, because the body continues to respond to the tiny, but potentially widespread, silicone particles. In many women who receive silicone breast implants, the macrophages keep accumulating month after month, year after year, like water that flows and collects from a valve that's never closed. As more cells arrive, the scar tissue becomes increasingly thicker, often creating a series of hard, painful lumps or overall hardening of the breast, in addition to the likelihood of changes in the physical contour of the breast itself. An overall immune-system response is once again triggered.

As stimulated antigen-processing macrophages migrate into the lymphatic channels, these cells soon enter the lymph nodes. Here, they interact with other immune cells, particularly T cell lymphocytes, causing the lymph nodes to enlarge and become repositories of "angry" immune cells. Views through a microscope have revealed a condition called *reactive hyperplasia*, which is an overgrowth of the lymph node resulting from reactions to environmental factors, including silicone.

Scientists agree that microscopic quantities of silicone reach the lymph nodes along with immune cells. But there is disagreement over what happens to these substances once they are in the nodes. Ultimately, silicone particles may be able to travel throughout the entire body. It is hypothesized that this may occur via the following process:

1. Lymph fluid goes into the chest in a tubelike collecting system called the thoracic duct.

2. This fluid and possibly the silicone particles themselves travel through the thoracic duct into the right side of the heart and the lungs.

3. Once it is past the lungs, the left side of the heart pumps the lymph and silicone particles out to the rest of the body. As a result of entering the bloodstream due to this sequence of events, silicone may trigger a bodywide immune-system response.

Should runaway stimulation of lymphocytes (B cells, helper T cells, and killer T cells) take place, a breakdown of the immune system, known as an autoimmune disease, may occur. Such a disorder may affect a single organ or many body parts. When an autoimmune disorder occurs, armies of invader-fighting cells are continually generated, which violently and mistakenly attack other sectors of healthy cells, breaking down the body piece by piece.

Whether internally or externally triggered, autoimmune disease results from the body's mistaken initiation of a devastating cellular blitzkrieg upon itself.

Rheumatic Reactions to Silicone

Many of the immune system responses reported by women with silicone breast implants are rheumatic in nature, which means that they affect the body's joints, muscles, and connective tissue, the material that holds together the very structure of the body.

Silicone exposure can affect the entire musculoskeletal system in numerous and serious ways. The manifestation and intensity of any given individual's health problem will vary: some severe, some mild or moderate, and some not at all. Clinical observations show, however, that when problems do manifest, they generally result initially from inflammation around the implants themselves.

As previously noted, inflammation is a normal aspect of the healing process, helping create an environment conducive to tissue repair and elimination of bacterial invaders. However, if these inflammatory conditions continue, "localized" rheumatic effects may become systemic.

For example, when a violent injury such as an ankle sprain occurs, the affected area swells up to immobilize the site and promote healing. This swelling, known as acute inflammation, involves the dispatch of a large force of bacteria-attacking neutrophils. Also directed to the affected area are *mast cells*, which release substances such as *histamine*—a chemical that expands blood vessels—into the tissue around the injury site to aid in the healing process. (Allergy sufferers are no doubt familiar with *antihistamines*, which block the effects of histamine to reduce swelling in sinuses and nasal passages.)

Since exposure to silicone in women with implants is often measured in years, unlike the acute, short-term inflammation of an injury, this long-term exposure can induce a far more problematic inflammatory condition, known as *chronic inflammation*. As its name implies, chronic inflammation is of long-term duration and involves proliferation of a wide variety of immune-system cells, including neutrophils, mast cells, macrophages, lymphocytes, and others. This type of inflammation takes hold in the presence of especially potent bacteria and certain viruses, as well as chemicals of low-grade toxicity—adding further support to the notion that silicone is far from an inert, "biocompatible" substance in the human body.

The immune system is an impressive, highly responsive, disease-fighting machine. When it is overstimulated or excited, however, a broad range of health disorders may occur.

Muscle Tissue

In women who have silicone implants, inflammation usually manifests itself first in various upper-body muscle tissues, stimulating the complaint of myalgia, or general muscle pain. Among the first muscles to fall victim to myalgia is the trapezius—the muscle that draws the shoulder back and up. Women afflicted by myalgia may feel tenderness, muscular stiffness, and pain in the upper part of the chest, neck, or upper back, or a combination thereof.

Irritation of the muscles is caused by the sheath of fibrous scar tissue that forms around the implant. By putting continuous pressure on the muscle, this scar tissue can also create a condition leading to permanent muscular spasm. Muscle stiffness and pain in the muscles of the upper back, such as the trapezius, may also be due in part to the increased weight of the breasts resulting from insertion of the implants. The combination of chronic inflammation, fibrous tissue formation, and increased muscular exertion required to support the implants often produces the effect of muscle pain in some women.

Other prime targets for silicone breast implant–related symptoms are the joints and the lymphatic system. Following the onset of muscle pain, tenderness, and tightness, there may be swelling and pain in the joints as a result of inflammation. Other inflammatory symptoms may include heat, redness, swelling, and fluid buildup in the affected joints.

Lymphatic System

Silicone that enters the lymphatic system leads to swelling of the lymph nodes, a problem that can occur throughout the body should silicone migrate beyond the area around the implant. Swollen glands in the chest, neck, underarms, and abdomen may result, along with other associated chronic flulike symptoms of low-grade fever (100° to 101°), fatigue, and pain in muscles and joints.

In some cases, production of lymphocytes may be so strongly induced that blockage of a lymphatic channel occurs. Depending on its location, this blockage could create serious problems, such as fluid collecting in the lungs. Further clinical studies are required to determine the extent to which the lungs may be a major target organ in silicone-associated connective tissue disease.

Autoimmune Diseases

The most serious conditions that result from the diffusion of silicone into the body are autoimmune disorders, whereby the body's immune system mistakenly and unceasingly attacks healthy cells, tissues, and musculoskeletal structures. (The natural causes of most of these diseases are not known, and many types of these diseases exist; there are approximately 100 forms of arthritis alone.)

The following is a brief summary of the autoimmune diseases that may be directly related to, or worsened by, silicone exposure, based on the clinical assessment of hundreds of USF patients. While each of these diseases also occurs in people who have not been exposed to silicone, the majority of patients with these illnesses (more than two out of three studied) have demonstrated mild to significant improvement following implant removal.

Rheumatoid Arthritis

Two to three times as many women as men suffer symptoms of this serious arthritic disorder, which include inflammation of the body's joints, notably the fingers, wrists, toes, ankles, and elbows. These joints may become painful, stiff, swollen, and, in severe cases, even deformed.

This condition may also lead to inflammation and weakening of the ligaments, tendons, and muscles around the affected joints. Sleep or other periods of prolonged physical inactivity are typically followed by increased stiffness and edema (fluid buildup) within joint tissues. Accompanying problems may include damage to peripheral nerves resulting in numbness, tingling, pain, or muscle weakness. Other areas that may become inflamed include the white of the eye (known as *scleritis*), the membrane around the heart (*pericarditis*), the spleen (*splenomegaly*), and the lymph nodes (*lymphadenopathy*).

The inflammation caused by rheumatoid arthritis may be intermittent in some patients and may resolve in others. The condition can lead to destruction of the afflicted joint or joints, leading in turn to varying degrees of joint deformity and disability.

Systemic Lupus Erythematosus

Inflammation is also the key symptom of this disease, but with lupus the target is connective tissue. Systemic lupus erythematosus affects nine times as many women as men, usually those of childbearing age, and appears to be more common in blacks, West Indians, and Chinese. In certain high-risk groups, the incidence may be as high as 1 out of every 250 women.

Discoid lupus erythematosus, the more common of the two versions of the disease, affects exposed areas of the skin. Characteristic symptoms start as a rash appearing as one or more red, circular, thickened areas of skin that turn into scars. These blotches may appear on the face, behind the ears, and on the scalp. Permanent hair loss may occur in affected areas.

Far more serious is *systemic* lupus erythematosus. This version of the disease affects many systems of the body, including the joints and kidneys. It causes a red, blotchy, butterfly-shaped rash on the cheeks and bridge of the nose, but no scarring. Other symptoms include feelings of malaise, fatigue, fever, loss of appetite, nausea, joint pain, and weight loss. Patients with systemic lupus also show a positive reading on an antinuclear antibody (ANA) test, indicating an overstimulation of their immune systems.

The *anemia of chronic disease*, a condition resulting from inefficient iron usage by the body, may also occur. Manifestations include neurological or psychiatric problems, kidney failure, pleurisy, arthritis, and pericarditis.

Lupus tends to run in families, and environmental factors such as sunlight and ingestion of certain drugs may trigger its appearance. *Drug-induced* lupus may be stimulated from exposure to various medications, most commonly heart drugs, such as quinidine and pronestyl, which are used for treating irregular heart rhythms. Symptoms of this version include onset of chronic fatigue, muscle and joint pains, fever, lung pain, and migraine headaches.

Scleroderma

Probably the worst of the rheumatic/autoimmune diseases, scleroderma is demonstrated by an increased growth of fibrous tissues of dermis, which is the layer of skin underneath the outer layer of epidermis. The result is a continual thickening of the skin. Twice as many women as men are victimized by this disorder, with symptoms usually appearing between the ages of 40 and 60.

The most common symptom of scleroderma is *Raynaud's phenomenon*, an extreme sensitivity of the hands and fingers to cold that can result in blanching and numbness or pain in the fingers. The skin may also tighten and become shiny, making it difficult to bend the fingers, open the mouth, and make other movements.

More serious scleroderma-related conditions ensue when the disease attacks the arteries, kidneys, lungs, heart, and gastrointestinal tract. Victims may experience difficulty swallowing, shortness of breath, heart palpitations, high blood pressure, joint pain, stiffness, and muscle weakness. In the most severe cases, there can be heart failure, respiratory failure, or severe hypertension and kidney failure leading to death. Progress of this disease is often rapid in the first few years; then it may slow down or even stop.

Fibromyalgia

A syndrome of musculoskeletal pain, stiffness, and easy fatigability, fibromyalgia (also called *fibrositis*) is a condition that occurs in women of childbearing age in 80 percent to 90 percent of cases. Generalized muscle pain and aching are the most common complaints.

Perhaps the most curious, and telltale, manifestation of fibromyalgia is that, despite the various symptoms reported by the patient, medical testing often fails to determine an objective problem. The only abnormal finding discerned in fibromyalgia patients, by and large, is the presence of numerous "tender points" in specific areas of the body that elicit pain when pressed.

Dermatomyositis

This rare condition involves inflammation of the muscles and skin that causes a skin rash and muscle weakness. Dermatomyositis can be fatal if it attacks the lungs or other organs. Two-thirds of the sufferers of this disease are middle-aged women.

The first manifestation of dermatomyositis is a red rash that appears on the bridge of the nose and cheeks, followed by a purple discoloration of the eyelids and sometimes a red rash on the knees, knuckles, and elbows. Muscles become weak, stiff, and painful, with the shoulders and the pelvis (where limbs join the trunk) most likely to be affected. The skin over these areas may feel thicker than normal, and the patient may experience nausea, weight loss, and fever.

Polymyositis is similar to dermatomyositis, but demonstrates no skin rash. Additional clinical data is needed to confirm a definitive connection between silicone exposure and these diseases.

Amyotrophic Lateral Sclerosis (ALS)

This motor neuron disease, also known as Lou Gehrig's disease, is extremely rare (about 1 to 2 cases a year per 100,000 people in the United States). It involves degeneration of nerves within the brain and spinal cord that control muscular activity. This incurable condition results in atrophy, or a wasting away, of the muscles and virtually always results in death.

First symptoms are usually a weakness in the hands and arms, and in some cases an involuntary quivering of small areas of muscle. Many of the afflicted also suffer from cramping or stiffness. The starting point of the symptoms may vary, but in virtually every case all four extremities are soon involved. Death usually occurs within two to four years, as the weakness progresses to the muscles of respiration and swallowing.

ALS usually affects people over 50 and is more common in men than women. About 10 percent of ALS cases run in the family. The only known treatment at this time is exercise therapy.

Multiple Sclerosis (MS)

This progressive disease of the central nervous system involves the destruction of *myelin*, the protective covering of nerve fibers in the brain and spinal cord. This degeneration results in symptoms ranging from numbness and tingling to paralysis and incontinence.

The severity of symptoms in MS varies considerably among those with the disease. It typically starts in early adulthood, subsides, then recurs years later. Spinal cord damage can cause tingling, numbness, or a feeling of constriction in any part of the body. The extremities may feel heavy and become weak. Stiffness sometimes occurs and, if the nerve fibers to the bladder are involved, the patient may become incontinent.

If there is damage to the white matter of the brain, the patient may suffer from fatigue, vertigo, clumsiness, muscle weakness, slurred speech, unsteady gait, blurred or double vision, and numbness, weakness, or pain in the face. These symptoms may occur alone or in various combinations, and last from several weeks to several months. In addition, injury may trigger a recurrence of symptoms after remission.

Silicone-Associated Connective Tissue Disease

How does a woman know whether she is suffering from any of these "traditional" autoimmune diseases or a silicone-induced version? Telling the difference is difficult even for rheumatologists who treat arthritis patients every day, since both types of disorders can involve various types of inflammation, overstimulation of the immune system, and similar types of pain. The chief distinction that can be made thus far is that silicone-induced disease usually begins with swollen lymph nodes and muscle pain in the chest around the implants, as well as in the upper back and neck. The pain then spreads into the shoulders and down the arms, and eventually becomes widespread in muscles and joints. The chronic fatigue gradually worsens.

In the previous chapters, we have offered our explanation of *how* silicone breast implants can cause silicone-associated connective tissue disease and *what* its symptoms are. Now we will move on to a critical examination of *why* implants were allowed to be put into women's bodies for 30 years without serious investigation. What went on in the R&D laboratories and marketing departments of breast implant manufacturers? What took place at the offices of the Food and Drug Administration? It's a complicated story—and the next chapter will show you how things happened.

Part II:
What Went Wrong?

Chapter 4

The Role of Manufacturers and the FDA in the Silicone Controversy

○ *The pain is so severe, I'll kill myself . . . .*

Betty, age 31, wanted to know what could be done about her small, flaccid breasts. So she wrote the American Society of Plastic and Reconstructive Surgeons and got a recommendation for a surgeon. When she met with her surgeon, he said he could give her "the breasts of an 18-year-old for the rest of her life." While Betty's breasts looked young after implantation, fifteen months after surgery they shifted to the sides and became hard and uncomfortable. She began having urinary tract infections that she couldn't shake. These difficulties were only a foreword to the impending assault on Betty's body.

Ten years after receiving her "youthful" breasts, severe fatigue, terrible back pains, insomnia, headaches, night sweats, neck and shoulder pain, aching legs, and irritable bowel syndrome became her constant companions. After having worked 12 hours a day, 6 days a week, as an insurance agent for years, Betty became so sick that she couldn't even get out of her car.

She was diagnosed with endometriosis and had a complete hysterectomy. Then she had a disc rupture in her back and was in such pain that she "didn't want to live anymore." Finally, after seeing 16 doctors during 15 years of suffering, Betty met a rheumatologist who saw the connection between her various symptoms and her breast implants. He enabled her to get disability compensation from her company and state, and she eventually made the difficult choice to have her implants removed. "I just knew it couldn't be anything else," she said. Recovery from her symptoms has been slow, but Betty has received a lot of support from her husband.

Women in Betty's support group echo one another's horror stories of doctors who didn't want to hear about their implant-related problems, doctors who told them that "they were going to be disfigured so bad when they take those implants out." She has also met women whose husbands have left them over the implants, including one woman Betty is sure died of silicone-induced disease. One of her friends once had silicone coming out through one of her nipples—and her doctor denied it even after he saw the evidence.

Manufacturers' Actions, Reactions, and Omissions During the "Implant Era"

For nearly three decades after the initial silicone-gel breast implantation in 1962, manufacturers and the FDA discussed the safety and efficacy of implants, both groups relying significantly on the medical profession, particularly plastic surgeons, for their observations and advice.

To date, implant manufacturers have responded to the silicone implant crisis primarily by taking legal measures to limit liability, rather than attempting to redress medical testing inadequacies and the ill effects these prostheses have had on untold thousands of susceptible women.

As an example, let's examine what occurred in *Teich v. FDA and Dow Corning*, the predominant player in the industry, in a 1990 case brought before the U.S. District Court for the District of Columbia. In the judge's memorandum opinion, it was cited that the plaintiff, a physician and consultant for Public Citizen, a private watchdog organization, had requested "a series of animal studies as well as a summary of consumer complaints about Dow Corning's breast implants," a request contested by the FDA, who claimed that the studies were privileged from disclosure as "confidential commercial information." Dow similarly resisted producing documents as privileged from disclosure. Wrote Stanley Sporkin, the U.S. District Court judge presiding on the case, "It is the decision of this court that the animal studies and the complaint summary are subject to disclosure and were wrongly withheld . . . ."[28]

The sheer volume of information that lawsuits, the FDA, the media, and organizations such as Public Citizen, the National Women's Health Network, the Command Trust Network, and others have brought to light regarding documents and testing results by implant manufacturers has revealed that company management ignored the accumulating evidence against silicone implants.

The record suggests that the reporting of adverse reactions to devices by manufacturers is often subpar; this has occurred with drugs as well. Similarly, it appears to many women and implant industry observers alike that manufacturers largely remained silent when it came to sharing any bad news about silicone implants.

Attesting to this point, a computer printout of breast implants returned to one manufacturer between 1979 and 1987 noted more than 1,200 citations of returned devices—due either to patient illness following implantation or rejection by the surgeon of a new prosthesis for one reason or another. In addition to product returns following explantation because of capsule formation, infection, rupture, or necrosis (poor blood flow to the breast resulting in tissue death), the report also noted units broken during insertion; bubbles, spots, or particles in the gel; cloudy, runny, or discolored gel; envelope inconsistency; calcification; fungal growth in gel; valve delamination; and leakage.[29] Was this common knowledge to patients? Given that silicone-gel implants were a multimillion-dollar-a-year industry, the steady flow of income may have made it easy for manufacturing executives not to notice anything except their bottom lines.

Did Gel Reformulation Create Problems?

It is the authors' opinion that the silicone-gel implants that appear to have prompted an increase in documented health and safety problems for women are those produced since approximately the mid-1970s, a time when reformulations were being made in implants by Dow Corning. These efforts were undertaken to develop more desirable prosthesis designs (with softer gel characteristics to adapt to the new, thinner-shelled jackets) to enable Dow to vie for market share in what was becoming an increasingly competitive breast implant marketplace.

At or about that time, Dow Corning Wright (a joint venture between Dow Chemical Company and Corning Inc.) was reported still to be the leading producer of silicone-gel breast implants, but according to a 1975 internal document the company's marketing objective was to "regain market share and slow down current Heyer Schulte momentum and potential McGhan [Medical Corporation] entry [into the market], i.e., prevent further market share erosion."[30]

Responding to this competition, Dow formed a Mammary Task Force (MTF), chaired by A. H. Rathjen, the man charged with the development and delivery to market of two new products: a low-profile, round prosthesis and a low-profile contour line.

The MTF met regularly—more than a dozen times between January and September 1975—and was apparently under strong pressure to meet its goals quickly. Much later the FDA and other industry investigators conducted analyses and suggested that in order to generate fast sales to hold their competitive position, Dow rushed its new products to market before they could be adequately tested—though this was officially denied years later by company officials. In an FDA document believed to have been prepared during 1990 (which reviewed and summarized Dow's internal memorandums from January 1975 through April 1987), the agency expressed strong concerns with "the apparent fast development and push to marketing this device had received in light of questions about lack of quality assurance specifications and safety tests" between February and May 1975.[31] Highlighting these ongoing product-development safety concerns, a brief excerpt of the FDA's commentaries, written by its personnel after reading Dow's 1975 Mammary Task Force paper trail, follows:

February 19, 1975

Dow memo: A notation is made that written specifications for [the new] envelope thickness still . . . do not exist.

FDA concern: "Why is manufacturing still continuing [without these specifications]?"

March 7, 1975

Dow memo: Human trials [on the new product] continuing . . . [while] quality of [the] envelopes [is] still being questioned.

FDA concern: "Additional [human] testing [is] still planned to continue [by Dow] in spite of concerns over quality and animal study results."

March 14, 1975

Dow memo: While proposals for completing envelope specifications are still being developed, 16,000-plus filled implants are [now in] stock.

FDA concern: "Where are the final specifications for [envelope] thickness?"

March 21, 1975

Dow memo: A 15 percent defect rate is noted: "This is the lowest sustained rate the plant has run." Reference is made [in Dow staff meetings regarding] what can be done to speed up the 90-day . . . test . . . so marketing can take advantage of [upcoming] regional meetings . . . to get the word out and start taking orders.

FDA concern: "This raises the question of previous defect rates and the amount of control there is over the manufacturing process."

March 26, 1975

Dow memo: A question is raised [by Dow staffers] regarding how an unsuitable lot [of new implants] got so far through quality control as to be filled [in preparation for release to market].

FDA concern: "What is the level of quality control?"[32]

These excerpts suggest that haste in the company's product development may have led to cutting corners regarding quality-control specification and safety testing. Public records of other internal Dow memos show that some of Dow Corning's staffers had expressed worries over what was happening, including questioning whether the less viscous gel being reformulated for the new implants posed a greater tendency to leak from the implant jacket.

In a series of memos from January to June 1976, Rathjen repeatedly called for more testing. His requests had followed the launch of the new products, given that the company was receiving some negative comments from surgeons regarding product performance. In January, Rathjen wrote, "We [had] better get going on a basic long range project [regarding] gel, its formulation, toxicology, etc. over and above what is now underway. The same goes for the envelope. The complaint report [we've just received from one plastic surgeon] is just one more flag!"[33] But apparently no action was taken.

In March, he wrote, "I think it would be embarrassing to Dow Corning . . . if we find [safety testing regarding gel migration] . . . left to a doctor in the field. If he were to come up with something detrimental, I think we ought to be prepared for it." Again, no internal action appears to have been taken. Then, in May, Rathjen attempted to arrange for research with an outside physician to conduct laboratory work in an effort to determine "[whether] there [is] something in the implant that migrates out or off the mammary prosthesis? Yes or No!" Was the research initiated? Again, it appears not. And finally, in June, he wrote, "I have proposed again and again that we must begin in-depth study of our gel, envelope, and bleed phenomenon. Capsule contracture isn't the only problem. Time is going to run out on us if we don't get underway." No apparent action was taken then either.

Though Rathjen's requests for testing seems to have gone unheeded, it does appear that company officials were worried about how such gel bleed might affect a plastic surgeon's sales pitch. In a May 13, 1975, memo, Dow engineer Tom Talcott, who headed the company's technical services and development group (and who quit the company the following year), sent an advisory memo to fellow staffers stating: "We are hearing complaints from the [sales force] about the demonstration [silicone implants] they are receiving. The general claim is that the units bleed profusely after they have been flexed vigorously.

. . . Please run appropriate testing when you receive these samples to determine if a bleed rate problem exists."[34]

Three days later, however, a memo was sent by Tom Salisbury, a marketing executive on the task force, which offered the following comments in response to Talcott's advisory:

> It has been observed that the new mammaries . . . have a tendency to appear oily after being manipulated. This could prove a problem with your [sales presentations to surgeons] where manipulation is a must.
>
> Keep in mind that this is not a product problem; our technical people assure us that the doctor in the [operating room] will not see any appreciable oiling on product removed from the package. The oily phenomenon seems to appear the day following manipulation.
>
> You should make plans to change demonstration samples often. Also, be sure samples are clean and dry before [sales presentations]. Two easy ways [to do this] while traveling are: 1) Wash with soap and water in nearest washroom, dry with hand towels; 2) Carry a small bottle of [cleaning fluid] and rag.[35]

What Did the Early Tests Show?

Before any material or medication can be studied in humans, the FDA requires that analysis for drug or device safety be conducted in animal subjects. The negative effects on animals are then evaluated, and only when findings register within certain acceptable guidelines may a manufacturer proceed to study its medical products on humans in "clinical trial" settings. (Adverse effects on animals are often indicators of potential problems, although effects on animals and humans may not always, and often do not, correlate.)

As a starting point, let's examine the findings of two Dow Corning reports. The first, dated February 7, 1975, as reported in the *New York Times*, was claimed to describe studies on rabbits showing "mild to occasionally moderate acute inflammatory reaction."[36] (In another report, dated March 6, 1975, 28 rabbits were tested with various injected gels and showed a "mild to moderately acute granulomatous inflammatory reaction.")[37]

Although these reactions were claimed in the Dow reports to be due to the trauma of the surgery itself rather than directly to silicone, the *Times* article went on to report that "eight women in Vancouver had already received [the new implants under development] in what the company described as a 'clinical experiment.' The company says the women were informed that the devices were experimental." The article further asserted that Dow files stated that "clinical [human] testing of sterilized mammary prostheses began February 3, 1975, four days before results from the animal tests were reported."[38]

At the time, Robert T. Rylee, vice president of Dow Corning Corporation and chairman of Health Care Businesses, reportedly claimed that the gel being used "was not a new material" and had already been well tested. Regarding the initiation of human testing of the new mammary prostheses prior to the evaluation of the animal data, Rylee said, "We intended it to be simultaneous [in humans and animals]."[39] It was not. Why?

In-house Memos

According to internal memoranda between officials of Dow Corning, some employees at the company had had concerns since the 1970s that the implants could leak or rupture.[40] In a 1978 memo, Dow Corning's technical director of health care, Robert R. LeVier, stated to other staffers:

> The 180-day rabbit gel implantation study [just completed] led to two conclusions based on the data:
>
> 1. The evidence . . . warrant[s] the conclusion that a hypothesis favoring efficacy in mammary augmentation . . . [or] reconstruction cannot be supported without further experimentation.
> 2. The evidence . . . is sufficient to raise a theoretical question concerning dissemination of gel or its components.[41]

Yet a 1992 *New York Times* article reported that "officials at Dow Corning maintain that the implants are safe, that most women who have them are delighted with them, and that the memorandums among the documents challenging company practices paint an inaccurate and incomplete picture." "This is a normal part of business activity," Dow health care business chief Rylee was quoted as saying, "people voicing their opinions, to help guide and direct the company." The *Times* went on to note, however, that Rylee "conceded that the company probably should have carried out some studies it did not to see whether there were more problems, such as inflammatory diseases caused by silicone that spreads throughout the body."[42]

However, almost 16 years to the day before the silicone implant story broke wide open, another Dow staffer was growing increasingly uncomfortable with product claims of safety. Amplifying Rathjen's feelings, 24-year veteran Dow engineer Thomas Talcott wrote the following words in a January 15, 1976, memo after receiving physicians' complaints about product-related problems (including possible leaked or bleeding gel that might migrate through recipients' bodies):

The general tone of [company reports given at a breast symposium] was one of disappointment that we are not #1 in the marketplace . . . [and] disappointment that two of our [implants] broke during augmentation surgery for the TV tape demonstrations.

During our task force assignment to get the new products to market, a large number of people spent a lot of time discussing envelope quality. We ended up saying the envelopes were "good enough" while looking at gross thin spots and flaws in the form of significant bubbles . . . .

When will we learn at Dow Corning that making a product "just good enough" almost always leads to products that are "not quite good enough"?[43]

Five months later, Rathjen noted in a memo the need for more research "to deal with the problem of capsular contracture," another problem of growing concern. "We are engulfed in unqualified speculation—nothing to date is truly quantitative or qualitative," he wrote.[44]

Later that year, Talcott reportedly "quit his job . . . in a dispute over the implant's safety."[45] Today, he serves as an expert witness on the subject of breast implants. Countered Dan T. Hayes, President and CEO of Dow Corning Wright (which included the breast implant subsidiary at the time), Talcott "left as a disgruntled employee. You've got to question to some degree his motives."[46]

According to another confidential memo, a Dow employee wrote to technical director Robert LeVier in March 1977, stating that he misled plastic surgeons when he told them that contracture/gel migration studies were under-way, in his own personal attempt to keep an important business relationship going.[47]

"Several of our customers, looking to us as leaders in the industry, asked me what we were doing," the marketing executive wrote. "I assured them, with fingers crossed, that Dow Corning . . . had an active [contracture/gel migration] . . . study underway. This apparently satisfied them for the moment, but one of these days they will be asking us for the results of our studies."[48]

In September 1983, a high-ranking Dow official related to his superiors that reports claiming implants do not leak or rupture were wrong. He wrote, "Only inferential data exists to substantiate the long-term safety of these gels for human implant applications . . . I must strongly urge [studies] to validate that these gels are safe. I feel this should be given top priority because of the volume of existing business, the extensive population of already implanted devices, and, especially, because [the company has not] indicated plans to obsolete this gel technology."[49]

We have reviewed three other Dow Corning documents written between 1980 and 1983—letters from surgeons and researchers as well as another internal memo. All note concerns of safety: one cites excessive gel bleed; the second refers to a collection of "data [that] suggests strongly that fibrosis and capsule contracture seen clinically may be an immunologically mediated phenomenon"; and the third reports a failed silicone implant in which the "patient had [a] considerable reaction . . . [which] I believe . . . proves the point that 'pure silicone' can cause severe foreign body reactions in susceptible individuals." This point was made by a surgeon in a 1981 letter to Dow Corning's Robert Rylee.[50]

"To put a questionable lot of mammaries on the market is inexcusable," noted a Dow employee in April 1980. "I don't know who's responsible for this decision, but it has to rank right up there with the Pinto gas tank."[51]

Lack of Testing Aired in Courtroom

According to a report published in *Business Week*, a lawsuit in 1984 against Dow Corning determined that the company "had committed fraud in marketing its implant as safe." In a post-trial ruling in which jurors awarded a Nevada woman $1.5 million in punitive damages, the article quoted U.S. District Judge Marilyn Hall Patel as writing that the company's own studies "cast considerable doubt on the safety of the product," which was not disclosed to patients. The judge upheld the jury's findings and said that the jury could conclude that Dow's actions "were highly reprehensible."[52]

The same article reported that Dow "totally disagreed" with the verdict, calling it "a highly charged, emotional piece of litigation." The following year, the company nevertheless changed its product literature to mention the possibility of immune-system sensitivity and silicone migration following rupture.

However, Dow Corning reportedly discounted the immune-system problem only two years later (though potential immune-system warnings remained in patient literature), reportedly saying it was linked to silicone of lesser purity than that used in its implants. Dow technical director LeVier had himself observed 9 years earlier that evidence existed that was at least "sufficient to raise theoretical questions concerning dissemination of gel." Dow Corning had then begun a program to replace ruptured implants and those removed when patients complained of adverse reactions, according to *Business Week*—all the time denying that the implants could cause such problems.

"Typically, the reaction [to silicone leakage] is benign," disputed Dow's Rylee. "It's picked up by the lymph system, transported around, and either excreted or stored." And in a 1992 article, the *Wall Street Journal* reported that "Dr. LeVier and other top Dow Corning officials continue to believe that, while the immune system question is a serious one, there isn't enough scientific evidence to prove the implants cause such maladies."[53]

There was no investigation of possible immune-system reactions to silicone by Dow until 1991 when a study appeared that the company reportedly claimed took two years to design. Back in 1985, a memo from Dow's business development specialist James Cooper regarding biosafety testing concerns noted that "a series of events [at the FDA] over the last 60 days" had prompted him to convey the following thoughts: the agency, in an apparent shift, was requiring *lifetime* animal testing for all new implant applications. "Taken to an extreme, this . . . [new] situation [at the FDA] is ominous [for us]," he wrote. "Most of our claims to date have been based on a two-year dog study. . . . However, a dog study must continue for seven years to qualify as lifetime testing. The materials used in [our] two-year dog study would not be approved under the lifetime test criteria." The study, performed by Dow Corning in 1968–70 by Food and Drug Research Laboratories, was based on four beagles that had been implanted with five materials. (It should be emphasized that the research lab's report cited "adverse effects" as including "fibrous tissue encapsulation and chronic inflammation" in one of the dogs.) Was it this very "study" the company depended upon for so many years to demonstrate biosafety?[55]

Dr. Norman Anderson, Associate Professor of Medicine, Department of Internal Medicine, Johns Hopkins Outpatient Center, and the chairperson of the FDA advisory panel investigating breast implants during this time, "characterized as astonishing the lack of directly relevant scientific studies of materials that Dow had sent to the FDA upon request," stated a January 1992 *New York Times* article. After reviewing a proverbial paper blizzard of 10,000 pages of Dow company submissions, Anderson found that none of the studies in animals had put silicone or implants in or under breast tissue. He reportedly claimed: "I find this omission a peculiar phenomenon which must be unprecedented in the history of medical device evaluation."[56]

Soon after, the late Representative Ted Weiss of Manhattan—who acted as chairman of a subcommittee of the Committee on Government Operations (which has jurisdiction over the FDA, and which investigated the safety of silicone implants)—was cited in another *New York Times* article as saying that Dow Corning's studies had been completely inadequate to answer even the most basic questions about silicone in the body, not to mention the long-term effects of having implants. Weiss's view (reported by the *Times*) was that only a handful of the women whose records were reviewed had been implanted for more than five years, while many complications take longer than that to develop. Weiss also cited documents that raised "serious questions about misbranding and scientific misconduct" by Dow Corning, and called for both the FDA and the Justice Department to investigate Dow Corning's conduct.[57]

Finally, negative publicity began to take its toll on Dow Corning—especially after more and more lawyers started sniffing blood. In December 1991, the company was ordered to pay $7.3 million in compensatory and punitive damages in the case of Mariann Hopkins, a California woman who claimed that the rupture of her implants and resulting silicone leakage led to the development of connective tissue disease. According to the *Wall Street Journal*, the federal court provided the money because Dow had concealed evidence linking ruptures in silicone-gel implants with autoimmune disorders. The company is appealing this decision.

Despite this and hundreds of other suits pending against Dow Corning, the company continued to assert in 1992 that its implants were safe—and that its tests proved that they were safe.

Dow Corning Communication Controversy

In December 1991, as mentioned in chapter 2, the FDA complained to Dow Corning after learning that at least some of the 40 women answering its nationally advertised 800-number information hotline for implants were misleadingly saying that the FDA had determined that the products were safe.[58] In response to these FDA complaints, Dow Corning shut down its toll-free service in January 1992.[59]

"Despite its self-avowed openness policy," a February 1992 *Wall Street Journal* article claimed that Dow Corning continued to "withhold from public view hundreds of internal documents related to the safety of silicone breast implants." The article reported that company attorneys were in the process of opposing the unsealing of safety and research memos entered as evidence in an eight-year-old suit in a San Francisco court.[60]

Finally, in March 1992, facing mounting negative publicity as well as legal and regulatory actions, Dow Corning got out of the implant business—at a cost of many millions of dollars to cover the shutdown.[61] The decision came just one week after Bioplasty Inc. had announced that it, too, would stop making implants. Bristol-Myers Squibb had stopped making polyurethane-coated gel implants the preceding summer. In 1991, approximately half a dozen companies had been marketing implants. By the time of Dow Corning's retirement, only two remained: McGhan Medical Corporation and Mentor Corporation.

As reported in *New Woman*, around that same time, Dow announced the creation of a $10-million fund for research and a program to give $1,200 to any woman with implants experiencing medical problems who wanted them removed but could not afford to do so.[62]

Polyurethane-Foam Implants

As discussed in previous chapters, polyurethane foam–coated breast implants were designed to help prevent capsular contracture. Foams were first used primarily in rebuilding the breasts of women who had undergone partial mastectomies, commonly performed in the 1960s. They were later used as a coating for implants, and by the late 1980s the foam-coated version was the most popular breast implant, with an estimated 200,000 having been sold in the United States alone. These implants were marketed under such brand names as Même, Natural Y, and Replicon.

Perhaps the key player in the successful marketing of this type of breast implant was Harold Markham. While working as a medical-supply salesman in Beverly Hills in 1970, he met and teamed up with John Pangman, the plastic surgeon who had invented the foam-covered implant. Markham first had the new silicone implants produced in volume by Heyer-Schulte Corporation, a California-based manufacturer of medical devices. But that company eventually lost faith in both the implant and Markham when Thomas Talcott, then director of materials research at Heyer-Schulte (and formerly at Dow), said that these implants sometimes caused a "gross inflammatory response" (though Markham's attorneys have countered that any such responses are short term).[63]

Talcott's assessment concerned James Rudy, the president of Heyer-Schulte, who later reportedly acknowledged in a *Wall Street Journal* article that no one at his company had ever checked the foam's chemical makeup. "I felt Markham claimed personal expertise he didn't have," Rudy was quoted as saying.[64] By the mid-1970s, the company had decided to stop making the polyurethane foam–coated implants due to growing concerns and later turned over its patent to Markham for free.

Markham has maintained that a study requested by his company in 1981 conducted by K. Gerhard Brand, a professor of medicine at the University of Minnesota, showed that 20 mice given miniature versions of the implants were evaluated over a 30-month period and showed no signs of cancer. However, Dr. Brand noted that the polyurethane cover might not have broken down in the mice, but surgeons had often reported such a breakdown in women. Again, direct correlations between animal and human data are dubious. Reported the *Wall Street Journal*, however: "There isn't any evidence that Mr. Markham did anything beyond Dr. Brand's study to learn the chemical makeup of his product." [65]

It turned out that the lining of these implants, described in company documents as the "patented Microthane interface system," was discovered by a University of Florida chemist to produce a dangerous substance known as TDA when it was broken down, a known animal carcinogen and a suspected human one. But the implant's lining actually had another name: Scott Industrial Foam, used in automobile air filters and carpet-cleaning equipment. When the manufacturer of the foam, Scotfoam Corporation, found out in 1987 that this material was being surgically implanted in women, it notified the implant manufacturer that the company was "shocked." "We do not recommend such uses," wrote Scotfoam product control manager Edward Griffiths. [66]

During a Florida liability lawsuit, the chemist who had analyzed the foam said that small amounts of TDA—or 2-toluene diamine—were produced in this breakdown. TDA is classified by the U.S. government as a hazardous waste and was banned for use in hair dyes in 1971; workers who handle it are advised to wear goggles, rubber gloves, and respirators. "TDA has been found in both the breast milk and urine of women with polyurethane-coated implants," reported the same *Wall Street Journal* article. [67] According to the FDA, about 10 percent of women with silicone-gel implants have those with polyurethane jackets. [68]

Markham is cited as "repeatedly claiming his products are safe." [69] Yet despite his claims, and strong ongoing sales at the same time, he may have seen trouble on the horizon; his foam implant business—then called Aesthetech—was acquired in 1988 by Surgitek, a Bristol-Myers Squibb Company. (Bristol-Myers reportedly declined to comment on whether it had been informed of any health-related questions about the foam when it made the acquisition.) And according to a report published in *Glamour*, not long before the company was acquired by Squibb, FDA officials decided to inspect the factory. Inspectors observed "employees blowing into the implants to test for inflation, and found a general lack of control over the sterilization process." [70] Markham, now in his early seventies, is retired.

It has been cited in press reports that Bristol-Myers continued to take the position that the TDA levels found in various tests were artificially created through the testing methods themselves. [71] Yet more recent tests designed for the manufacturer have also been claimed to note that the foam degraded into TDA. After the FDA issued a request for safety data, Bristol-Myers voluntarily withdrew the product from the market, avoiding the more serious investigation faced by manufacturers of silicone-gel implants.

Roadblocks to Recognizing Silicone-Induced Disease

- Animal studies that were poorly designed, and that lacked relevance and relation to humans.

- Premature marketing of implants, prior to long-term and autoimmune safety data collection and analysis.

- Too much dependence on surgeons for negative product-performance reports, resulting in little feedback; some information that was made available to manufacturers from the FDA was not passed along, some patients have claimed.

- Surgeons depended too heavily on manufacturers to advise them on what to expect regarding possible problems; when some surgeons told manufacturers of complications, little action was taken by the manufacturers.

- The industry withheld key research findings regarding connections between implants and autoimmune disorders from medical experts, peer-review literature, and regulatory agencies.

- Ineffective study protocol: many studies were carried out on too few women, addressed too few side effects, and were conducted over too short a period of time; some tests even evaluated implants in sites other than the breasts.

- Manufacturers responded slowly to FDA data demands, even though they knew safety data would eventually be demanded based on new FDA mandates, and were given two-and-a-half years' advance notice; when the date of submission finally came, adequate data was still not provided or available. Additionally, data presented at a November 1991 conference was judged by the General and Plastic Surgery Devices Panel of the FDA to be inadequate in areas of implant rupture, gel bleed and migration data, chemical information on solid silicone and liquid silicone gel, toxicity/bioreactivity data (including immune system, cancer, and birth defect studies), effects on tumor detection with mammography, psychological benefits of implants, and other areas.

Since the first silicone-gel implant, Dow Corning alone has sold over 850,000 implants, implanted in some 600,000 women.[72] But unlike automobiles that can be recalled before people are hurt due to manufacturing defects, implants that cause women problems can be removed only at great cost—and usually after great suffering with silicone disease. The rise and fall of the silicone breast implant is not the result of the manufacturers alone, however; the FDA played a big role as well.

FDA Regulation During the Implant Era

The Food and Drug Administration is not comprised of scientists who sit in labs testing experimental drugs and medical devices. The agency does no testing of its own; mostly, it reviews existing data or creates panels of experts who examine other studies, interpret their validity, translate the findings, and make judgments about whether a product is safe for use by the public.

This lack of direct involvement in the research end of product analysis is one reason why the approval process for new drugs and medical devices in the United States takes many years. In the case of silicone gel, the FDA relied to a great extent on test results submitted by manufacturers and was thus at the mercy of these tests' validity. Such evidence frequently takes many months or years to be gathered and provided to the FDA, thus limiting the agency's ability to provide timely protection of the public against an unsafe product.

The fact that the vast majority of women receiving implants were pleased with the results also made implants an unlikely target for investigation. For many years, it seemed that implants were loved by everyone—patients, doctors, and manufacturers. But that was before the reality of silicone disease was brought into sharper and sharper focus.

Breast Implants Bypassed Approval Process

The long approval period typical for virtually all medications and devices—except in the case of "orphan drugs," or those experimental pharmaceuticals deemed for compassionate use, such as in the investigational treatment of people with the AIDS virus—adds cruel irony to the virtually instant acceptance of silicone-gel breast implants after their invention in the early 1960s. While many women believed that what was being implanted into their bodies had been given the FDA's approval, in truth the implants had slipped through a strange regulatory loophole.

Regulation of drugs in the United States became much tougher in the early 1960s after the travesty of thalidomide, a drug taken by pregnant women which caused severe birth defects. However, while medical devices were meant to be more strictly regulated, along with drugs—they are to this day evaluated separately and with a different set of rules by the FDA—devices were stricken from the new regulation bill passed in 1962. This quirk occurred just in time to render the FDA powerless to make judgments about the new silicone-gel breast implants.

It was not until 14 years later, in 1976, that the FDA was granted the authority to regulate medical devices. However, this change in policy applied only to *new* devices. Breast implants, which had been in use for years in hundreds of thousands of women, were "grandfathered" by the FDA; that is, their safety was assumed because they had been used on an ongoing basis for years without demonstration of health risk. Safety data *was* asked for by the FDA; however, manufacturers were given many years to get together such information. Essentially, this grandfather designation by the FDA was a *lack of disapproval for silicone implants rather than a genuine approval of safety.*

In 1978, FDA scientists recommended that breast implants be put in a category that would require proof of their safety. For some reason, however, an early panel formed to evaluate the issue didn't require such proof at that time. The FDA moved toward the reclassification of implants again in 1982, this time placing them preliminarily into Class III, meaning that they were deemed to pose "a potentially unreasonable risk of injury." But due to the grandfather statute, safety data wouldn't be submitted for agency review for nearly a decade. The silicone implant safety studies thus slipped through one hole in the regulatory net after another. Stated Dr. Sidney M. Wolfe, director of the Public Citizen Health Research Group in a November 9, 1988, letter to former FDA Commissioner Frank Young: "You must explain why six and one-half years [have] elapsed before finalizing the FDA's January 19, 1982, proposal to require Dow and other companies making silicone gel breast implants to submit safety data. Your agency negligently did not finalize this regulation until June of this year."[73]

FDA Aware of Cancer Concerns with Foam-Coated Implants

In addition to various previously cited health issues, another letter from Public Citizen, this time in August 1989 to Congressman John Dingell, Chairman of the House Oversight and Investigations Subcommittee, charged that FDA officials knew in the 1980s that there were problems associated with polyurethane foam–covered implants and failures to report adverse patient responses—again, long before regulatory action was taken:

The plastic surgery community has conceded that there are significant problems with the polyurethane-covered implants, and several of its members have so testified in numerous product liability cases brought against manufacturers. In fact, we know of at least 35 lawsuits which have been brought against the manufacturer of the "natural Y" over the last 18 months . . . ."

[Further], the FDA conducted an inspection of Cooper Surgical/Aesthetech . . . its investigator found the company did not submit information on at least 11 incidents of silicone breast prosthesis failure that should have been reported . . . .

To our knowledge, the FDA has not initiated criminal prosecutions or injunctions against . . . companies . . . found by the FDA's own investigators to have illegally withheld reports . . . of serious injuries . . . or delayed sending those reports to the FDA."[74]

By 1985, the increasing prevalence of implant-related problems reported to the FDA led it to request more accurate information from manufacturers on their products' safety. But it wasn't until June 1988 that the FDA finally notified manufacturers that it was asking them to provide premarket approval information—the kind of scientific data that manufacturers of any new product would have to provide. However, the FDA gave the implant makers yet another 30 months to submit their data!

Could the FDA Have Done More?

Both consumer groups and numerous federal officials have raised questions about whether the FDA has enough power to protect the public from dangerous drugs and devices. Recent medical tragedies involving silicone breast implants, a popular sleeping pill, and a commonly used sedative, for example, clearly show that the public is often the last to find out about dangerous side effects.

In his memorandum opinion referred to earlier in this chapter, Judge Stanley Sporkin had this to say about the FDA:

In fact, Congress specifically empowered the FDA [in 1976] to require the submission of safety test results. Logically, this means that the agency would certainly be permitted to require research materials as part of its rulemaking procedure . . . .

The FDA argues that although it is empowered to promulgate a regulation requiring such submissions, this does not change the fact that it has not yet promulgated one for silicone breast implants, and therefore it is dependent upon voluntary submissions . . . . The agency has [thus] done little, if anything, to implement this extremely important and necessary authority for over 13 years.

To use this now as an excuse for continued ineffective regulation is nothing less than *chutzpah* being elevated to new heights.[75]

Here are some of the key factors that limit the FDA's power to protect the public:

1. Virtual impossibility of product recall

Unlike a car with defective brakes that can be pulled back into the dealer, many medical devices such as implants are integrated into a person's body and involve cost and risk to remove. And damage, once done, may not be reversible.

2. Lack of doctors' compliance

Doctors are not obligated to practice medicine on the basis of FDA opinion. The way the FDA gets into the physician's pocketbook, however, is by disallowing a specific Medicare-reimbursable labeling on a drug, device, or procedure. Without insurance or Medicare reimbursement, few patients can afford to take advantage of the medical advance, and so it dies right there.

3. No law-making capability

The FDA cannot create legislation to dictate behavior. It can only make recommendations, and has to rely on other government bodies to pass laws necessary to uphold its policies.

4. No subpoena power

Most federal agencies are allowed to obtain drug-company documents when suspicions are aroused—but not the FDA. For example, data that resulted in the FDA's ban of implants in early 1992 had been sitting for years in Dow Corning's files. These files had been disclosed to trial lawyers eight years before, but a court agreement had kept them confidential. Their lack of subpoena power means the FDA can only threaten criminal prosecution by the Justice Department. The FDA was very dependent on manufacturers abiding by the honor system—a dubious method of fact gathering, given manufacturers' vulnerability to, and fear of, lawsuits.

5. Diversion of research money to other areas

Both the FDA and the National Institutes of Health (NIH) have tended to focus on more exotic avenues of research than implants. This may reflect the desire of scientists who prefer to be on the ground floor of exciting new discoveries rather than analyzing old products. Also, research funds often come from manufacturers seeking new products that can build company profits—a source hardly available in the case of implants.

6. Antiregulatory government climate

We live in the shadow of deregulation left us during the Reagan years. This pro-business, anti-interventionist legacy has taken the bite out of investigations into many dubious products.

○ *A lot of women are too embarrassed to go to court . . . .*

Sybil Goldrich suffered an implant rupture that spread silicone to her ovaries, uterus, and liver. But a judge dismissed her lawsuit, saying that she had waited too long to file after her first problems appeared. "They say I should have known earlier that the implant caused problems," Ms. Goldrich was quoted as saying in the *New York Times.* "That's a little strange, given that the FDA doesn't seem to have been able to establish the problems very quickly."

Today, as head of the Command Trust Network, an advocacy group for women with breast implants, Ms. Goldrich helps women arm themselves for the arduous litigation battle against implant manufacturers. Meanwhile, she is appealing the dismissal of her own case—and fighting the manufacturers' demand to make her pay up to $75,000 of their court costs.[76]

Most of the key events in the FDA's hunt for the truth regarding silicone's effects on implanted women have occurred since 1988. The following is a basic chronology of events leading to the current FDA stance.

June 1988: FDA Designates Implants As "Unproven"

Based on data examined regarding the occurrence of allergic reactions, lymphadenoma, morbidity, and gel migration, the FDA gave silicone-gel implants a Class III rating, indicating that the safety of the implants remained unproven. The FDA also indicated that available data did not show implant-related health risks beyond the usual complications related to implantation and surgical procedures. Score this one a tie: Women: 0, Manufacturers: 0. The "unproven" rating obligated the manufacturers to do nothing.

November 1988: Advisory Panel Provides Guidelines on Data Gathering

A General and Plastic Surgery Devices Advisory Panel recommended to the FDA what information should be asked for in a regulation that would call for Pre-market Approval (PMA) applications. As a result of information presented at this meeting, the panel recommended that the FDA and the American Society of Plastic and Reconstructive Surgery should conduct a review of all existing national and international registries of breast implants. Data would be gathered on all known clinical and preclinical risks, including carcinogenesis and "immune disorders." This meeting was the first time that immune disorders were mentioned in advisory panel recommendations.

May 1990: FDA Lists Autoimmune Disease as Possible "Significant Risk"

The FDA announced its intention to require PMAs for silicone-gel implants and described potential benefits and risks. Based on the review recommended by the 1988 panel, the agency included "autoimmune disease/immunological sensitization" as a possible risk. Also listed were capsular contracture, leakage and migration, infection, interference with early tumor detection, degradation of foam-covered implants, carcinogenicity, teratogenicity (birth defects), and calcification.[77]

The agency observed that many of those commenting on the possible connection between silicone and autoimmune disorders claimed that the number of reported cases of such diseases among implanted women was no greater than the incidence in the general population. The FDA rejected these opinions, however, saying that the difference in autoimmune illness frequency between the two groups was not clear and therefore required further investigation.

December 1990: Congressman Weiss Blows Whistle on Silicone-Related Problems

A Congressional hearing was held to determine whether the FDA was adequately protecting patients from the dangers of silicone-gel breast implants. The late Representative Ted Weiss, Democrat of Manhattan, who chaired the subcommittee conducting the inquiry, was outspoken in his criticism of how the FDA had handled the implant issue. He stated that FDA representatives had not regulated implants as they should have, and that serious medical complications had befallen implanted women for many years. The FDA responded by saying that the type of research Weiss was proposing would cost many millions of dollars annually to conduct, and that such funds were not available. Weiss also raised concerns about the efforts and motivation of the FDA, contending that the agency had not effectively addressed many serious implant issues.[78]

In a letter to the FDA commissioner, Weiss wrote that "very serious scientific concerns about the polyurethane implants were obvious in FDA internal documents for several years . . . . I fear that some at the FDA became more concerned about the reputation of the manufacturer than informing the public." Weiss also reportedly asserted that the FDA had issued a press release with misleading information about the foam-coated implants. The release stated that the foam in these implants "might degrade" into TDA, even though FDA scientists had found it definitely did degrade. Weiss went on to say that the FDA did not make enough of an effort to get this information about TDA to implant recipients who needed it most, such as pregnant women or those who were nursing infants. "American women deserve better treatment," Weiss wrote.[79]

February 1991: FDA Sponsors Conference on Silicone in Medical Devices

Due to an increasing number of reports of adverse reactions to medical devices containing silicone, the FDA sponsored a conference; much of the discussion focused on immunotoxicity and autoimmune disease.

Findings presented included information showing antibody and cell-mediated immune responses to silicone-gel breast implants. Also demonstrated was a case series in which 12 women with connective tissue disease experienced varying amounts of relief following implant removal. Dr. John Varga of Jefferson Medical College and Dr. Steven Weiner, a Los Angeles–based clinician, both presented data at the FDA meeting that focused on the possible connection between silicone-gel implants and immune disorders, reviewing the results of several case studies involving from 1 to 15 women with implants. These patients were seen to have symptoms of connective tissue disease, including chronic myalgias, arthralgias, and arthropathies. The speakers commented, however, that a cause-effect relationship could not be conclusively proven from these studies alone.[80]

Upon reviewing with an independent panel some 10,000 pages of submitted data, the FDA decided that there was still not enough evidence to show that silicone-gel implants were safe.

April 1991: Manufacturers Required to File PMAs

The FDA published a ruling that required manufacturers of silicone gel–filled breast prostheses to file PMAs within 90 days, by July 9, 1991. The FDA also encouraged further research into the possible link between autoimmune disease or connective tissue disease and implants. After submission of the PMAs, the FDA was to evaluate the data and decide within 180 days whether the implants were sufficiently safe for use.

July 1991: PMA Applications Lack Safety Assurances

After receiving scientific data from only four of the seven manufacturers of silicone-gel breast implants—Mentor, McGhan Medical Corporation, Dow Corning Corporation, and Bioplasty Inc.—the FDA found that the information submitted was not sufficient for agency scientists to establish that implants were safe and effective; it was also noted that the data was insufficient.[81] This amplified the FDA's previous concerns, an agency background information report noted, particularly about the possible relationship between the implants and autoimmune disorders.

September 1991: FDA Requires
More Accurate Risk Information

The FDA sent letters to manufacturers requesting complete reports on both animal and human studies relating to the effects of implants and silicone. Manufacturers were also notified that their PMAs would be presented at an upcoming meeting of the General Plastic Surgery Devices Panel.

At this time, the agency issued a requirement to manufacturers to supply to plastic surgeons accurate data on the risks associated with breast implants, and requested that doctors, in turn, give this data to patients considering implant surgery. The manufacturers were given 30 days to provide this information.

The agency called for the "dissemination of information on risks" for both silicone and saline implants "to women considering having the devices implanted," and for the information to be "written so as to be easily comprehended to . . . patients and . . . provided . . . prior to scheduling implantation," so patients could consult with their physicians about risks. The FDA also provided manufacturers with "patient risk information sheets," which they encouraged manufacturers to print and distribute to physicians for dissemination to patients.

November 1991: FDA Panel Claims
Safety Data Incomplete

At a meeting of the General and Plastic Surgery Panel, the FDA concluded that the immunological effects of silicone-gel implants had not been adequately tested. In fact, some of the manufacturers had provided no scientific data whatsoever.

A total of 22 consumer groups and 60 implant patients testified at the proceedings. Taking the pro-implant position were the American Cancer Society, Why Me? (a support group), plastic surgery professional groups, and the American Medical Association.

Following testimony from FDA scientists and implant manufacturers, the committee concluded that the four manufacturers had not provided adequate information on the chemical properties of implant materials, mechanical and physical properties of the implants, frequency of adverse effects such as rupture and contracture, the extent to which implants mask tumor detection during mammography, and risks of cancer or immune disorders.

Data presented by certain firms was reportedly deemed inadequate even to support pre-market approval documents previously submitted to FDA. And although one manufacturer presented a large number of classic animal immunology studies, the FDA noted that there was "no universally accepted animal model . . . for the induction of autoimmune diseases." It was further noted that only human clinical studies of these devices in the body could determine whether there was in fact an association between the implants and autoimmune disease. This data was not gathered.

The panel chairperson, Dr. Elizabeth Connel of Emory University School of Medicine, pointed out that the panel did not find evidence that the implants were unsafe, but rather that there was not enough evidence shown about implant risks and benefits. Nevertheless, the panel voted unanimously to advise the FDA that implants served a need regarding the public health and should continue to be available while manufacturers gathered additional data. It recommended that implants could temporarily remain available to the public as long as three restrictions were met:

1. A National Implant Registry was to be established to track implant patients.

2. An informed consent document was to be issued to each patient.

3. A one- to three-year timeline for submission of safety data to FDA was established.

The FDA gave manufacturers 30 days to provide adequate patient information on implants, after which time any implant not providing such disclosure would be labeled as misbranded (which could lead to judicial actions). The agency said that it would complete its review of manufacturers' data and make a decision on their use by early January 1992.

FDA Commissioner David A. Kessler called the breast implant issue one of the most troubling he had to deal with in his post. He vowed that the FDA would require manufacturers to provide all the information needed to answer safety questions on silicone-gel breast implants, both for women who have implants and for those who might want them in the future.

January 1992: FDA Requests Ban on Silicone Implants

On January 6, Kessler declared a moratorium on the use of silicone-gel breast implants pending review of additional information about them. He said that the FDA's General and Plastic Surgery Devices Panel—the same panel that had met in November 1991 to review information about implant safety—would evaluate the new data and reconvene within the next 45 days to make new recommendations. Speaking for the FDA, Kessler stated: "We cannot assure the safety of this product."

Doctors were requested to stop using silicone breast implants, and all manufacturers to stop supplying them. Saline gel–filled breast implants were not included in the moratorium.

The FDA also recommended against routine mammograms to detect "silent" rupture of implants, and stated that other methods of rupture detection were still in the experimental stage and not necessarily reliable.

Data from Rheumatologists and Lawsuits Put Implants Under Fire

The key motivators for the moratorium were recent reports from some rheumatologists who were increasingly convinced of a link between implants and inflammation of joints and connective tissue, plus material from the files of one breast implant company that had come to light in legal proceedings.

There were also new concerns that some pre-1985 implants may not have been tested properly and had significant problems with leakage. Robert Rylee of Dow Corning reportedly disagreed with the FDA commissioner's action, but did agree to comply.[82]

Kessler made it clear in his statement at the time that the FDA was not opposed to breast implants. He recommended that women without problems with their implants not have them removed, but those who did should consult with their doctors. Obviously, the desire for hard-core information about implants was widespread; about 30,000 women had already called an FDA hotline set up to answer questions about silicone breast implants.

Some scientists argued that the moratorium was counterproductive to data gathering, because it allowed only a retrospective study of previous implant recipients. They said that such a study didn't allow the total control of parameters, variables, or subjects afforded by a designed study—thus limiting the value of its findings. Of course, since the FDA is not a legislator, none of its recommendations related to the moratorium were legally binding. However, virtually all parties involved agreed to comply.

April 1992: Implants Made Available for Reconstruction

The FDA lifted the total moratorium it had declared in January by announcing that implants would now be available for those who qualified for an "urgent need" category, as well as those taking part in long-term clinical protocol studies. Since the protocols were limited to a certain number of women, this policy made it unlikely for many women who wanted to enlarge their breasts to get silicone implants. The trials also required participating patients to fill out a very detailed consent form.

The moratorium was lifted in three stages:

1. Implants were made available to women who needed them most: those whose breast reconstruction had begun before the moratorium with placement of a temporary tissue expander and who were awaiting permanent implants, and those whose implants had ruptured.

2. Over a period of several months, clinical studies would be coordinated that were open to breast cancer patients and to women who had suffered serious trauma to a breast, or a disease or congenital disorder that caused breast abnormality.

3. More intensive research studies would be opened up to a limited number of women, those who wanted implants both for reconstruction and for cosmetic purposes. (This was the only avenue open to women who wanted implants for breast enlargement.)

The FDA estimated that, due to limited enrollment for studies, the yearly total of breast augmentation patients with silicone implants would drop to 2,000 or perhaps as little as even a few hundred women. The annual number of "urgent need" patients was approximated at 5,000 to 8,000 women, almost all of them cancer patients who had undergone mastectomies.

Kessler noted that all women enrolled in the studies would be monitored for years and informed of potential risks, and would have to give consent to receive the implants. Physicians who enrolled women in the studies were obligated to certify that saline implants would not be a satisfactory alternative.

The FDA claimed that the goal of the studies was to help answer questions about the frequency of rupture and leakage, frequency of side effects such as hardening of the skin around the implant, and the extent to which implants interfere with mammography.

The Right Choice

Since its recommendation for clinical trials with silicone implants, the FDA has come under attack by some experts who feel that a potentially risky product shouldn't be available to *anybody*, willing guinea pig or otherwise. On the one hand, the FDA is responsible for the protection of citizens against devices and drugs that may cause them harm. On the other, some women feel that they're being treated unfairly—that all women who are informed of the risk should have the right to choose for or against having implants.

Who has the right to determine who can take a health risk and who cannot? We smoke cigarettes that have warnings about lung cancer and birth defects to unborn children. We drink alcoholic beverages that we know can damage our bodies. Does a silicone-gel breast implant fall into this category? Is it a product that should simply be available to everyone willing to take the risks? Until the absolute risk factors are known, women who opt to experiment with silicone implants are playing a dangerous game, because no one can predict the outcome.

Women have been both grateful and impatient over the FDA's handling of the silicone implant issue. The administration under David Kessler got many vital findings about implants into the public arena. Many claim that previous FDA administrations failed to move in a timely manner to search for the truth about silicone and to get manufacturers to provide requisite and relevant safety data. Other FDA-related issues include the following:

- Numerous doctors—notably plastic surgeons—have maintained that the FDA withheld important scientific evidence from medical practitioners needed to make decisions about medical care.
- Others have claimed that the FDA often followed a "wait-and-see" policy regarding the implant saga. Much of its activity, which should have begun much sooner, had been spurred by the lawsuits against implant manufacturers.

- While discussions among the FDA and advisory panels about breast implants from 1978 to 1983 focused on gel bleed, silicone migration, fibrous capsule contracture and calcification, teratogenesis, hematoma, displacement of the implant, interference with tumor detection and postoperative lactation, and carcinogenesis, none of these discussions explored the possible connection between silicone exposure and immune disorders.

As of the spring of 1993, Dow Corning has changed direction and has hired new management, including CEO Keith McKennon and Medical Director Myron Harrison, M.D., M.P.H. In personal discussions, the authors have been advised that Dow Corning's executives are now seeking to achieve, finally, a clear understanding of the silicone controversy and to help resolve it with scientific studies—be they ultimately favorable to the company or not.

Were patients told the truth? Truth can be, and often is, a relative term. Manufacturers, patients, plastic surgeons, rheumatologists, the FDA, the public, watchdog organizations, the media—each group has its own version of the silicone story. Hence the same findings are interpreted by one group as confirming the dangers of silicone gel, and by another as inconclusive. Only definitive epidemiologic studies—now in process—will prove the issue one way or another. It is presently unclear how long this process will take.

Especially important in the quest for truth about implants is the plastic surgeon—an often-attacked player whose actions during the silicone crisis will be examined in the next chapter.

Chapter 5

How Much Did
Plastic Surgeons Know?

The doctor told me I wouldn't have any problems, and that they'd be there for
life . . . .

Sandra had a bilateral mastectomy at age 36, in 1986. Her surgeon
inserted tissue expanders into her breasts to stretch the skin, followed
by implantation of polyurethane-coated breast implants in 1987. Bleeding and oozing from her breasts began almost immediately and continued for four straight weeks.

When her surgeon had her return for the separate procedure
required to rebuild the nipples, Sandra's breasts had already begun to
harden. She was told that if she massaged them, they would get soft
again. So she did—nevertheless her breasts became rock-solid.

There soon followed a series of physical traumas: urinary tract
infections, burning sensations in her chest, and fevers that wouldn't go
away. Her doctor told her it was just a virus, yet her illness was still
going strong after eight weeks of treatment. One minute she would feel
fine, the next she would be on fire with a temperature of 103°.

Sandra's husband, unable to cope with her physical devastation and
emotional needs, he left her. She had no health insurance and was
rapidly going broke. Every week she was labeled with new syndromes:
Epstein-Barr virus, then Graves' disease, then something else. She felt
as though medications were coming at her from all angles, but the drugs
did nothing but drain her savings while offering no relief to her disease-
riddled body. Finally, when a chronic bronchial condition wouldn't
clear up, she was hospitalized and put on oxygen for seven days, at the
staggering cost of $12,000. She later developed a serious thyroid
condition, and her weight plummeted to 80 pounds.

Eventually, Sandra's doctor sent her to a rheumatologist, who
diagnosed her condition as lupus and told her that it might be due to her
implants. A lung specialist performed a bronchoscopy—an examination
of the bronchi of the lungs through a tube—and found that they were
filled with silica particles, a condition common in coal miners. Following implant removal in 1992, Sandra had a lung biopsy that detected
emphysema. She has never smoked a day of her life.

Sandra was fortunate to get disability compensation, and just in
time; she is now on a breathing machine at home. "I can't go out to a
restaurant or anything . . . can't even try to enjoy a decent meal," she
said. "I cough and gasp for breath all the time." Sandra's husband has
returned and lives with her again. Today he admits that he was wrong

89

to have pushed his wife into having the breast reconstruction. After almost losing her forever—and being unable to cope with the horrors of Sandra's medical problems—today he no longer cares whether or not she has breasts. His and her concerns have stretched far beyond that issue.

Plastic surgeons say they work hard to understand their patients' motivations when they inquire about breast augmentation. They look for motives that might be internal rather than external in nature. Self-esteem issues versus attracting a mate, for example. "It's sometimes hard to separate the two [motivations, however,] since where do those inner drives come from but the values we place on what everyone else thinks?" said Dr. Don La Russa, a plastic surgeon at the University of Pennsylvania.[83] Women who believe that implants alone will change their lives are regarded by surgeons as poor candidates for cosmetic augmentation due to their emotional profile, and many are therefore dissuaded from the procedure. Yet for years, all women who could afford the operation had an option. Don't like your breasts? Get new ones. The risks are slight and the benefits enormous, the promotion suggested. Make your body look great now.

According to an article in *Mother Jones*, about 750,000 women elect to have cosmetic surgery of some kind each year.[84] And as this business has grown, so too has the number of plastic surgeons. Said Dr. Jane S. Zones, a University of California medical sociologist, "the supply of plastic surgeons is growing ten times faster than the population."[85] Dr. Zones is a board member of the National Women's Health Network and also served as the consumer representative on the FDA's advisory panel that eventually recommended restricting the use of silicone breast implants.

To date, few plastic surgeons have gone on the record to express a definitive opinion on the validity of silicone-associated connective tissue disease. "The vast majority of women I see are ecstatic that they've had augmentation surgery," said a Florida plastic surgeon who would comment only on condition of anonymity. "As a matter of fact, when this whole scare came up, most of my patients asked me about it. My response was, if you're really concerned, take the implants out. But that's the last thing they'll have done.

"Whether it's safe or not, whether they were given the right information or not, whether there's such a thing as silicone-induced diseases, I don't know," the surgeon explained. "At this point, I feel there is not enough scientific evidence to state categorically that there is such a disease entity. I'm not going to state it doesn't exist; I'm just saying there isn't enough scientific evidence to convince me that it does."

Many plastic surgeons are less open-minded. Still others will admit (only off the record) that because they live in the world of plastic surgeons, they do not want to commit "political suicide" by taking a position that is at odds with that of the majority of their colleagues. In the summer of 1991, the American Society of Plastic and Reconstructive Surgeons "hit the panic button and began a multi-million-dollar lobbying campaign financed by assessing its members $1,050 each," reported the *Minneapolis Star Tribune*.[86] The ASPRS also was noted to ask its members "to recruit patients who could help make the case in Washington." The result: 400 implanted patients of different ages and backgrounds from 37 states came to Washington in October 1991 to voice their position. The surgeons who had organized the event asserted that implant use should be a personal decision, not the government's. Yet only happy patients were invited. Why not those women who were made ill as well? That's not a balanced presentation: that's lobbying. Why not put that lobby money back into the needed research on the medical and scientific issues? The plastic surgeons' money went to promote freedom of choice, not to determine product safety.

Today, the ASPRS continues to build up its fight against anti-implant publicity. According to a *Wall Street Journal* article: "The society has imposed the $1,050 levy on its members to raise a war chest of $3.9 million over the next three years; so far, it plans to spend about one-eighth of that on research and the rest for lobbying." Observed Dr. Zones, "The ASPRS [has] operated like a commercial enterprise rather than a collegial medical society." [87]

Yet this use of funds "has [also served to] enrage some plastic surgeons, who fear that responding to health concerns with an expensive lobbying campaign demeans the profession," said the *Journal*.[88] Apparently, the ASPRS is focusing primarily on protecting its own image—and not on the well-being of the patients of plastic surgeons who claim they are in need of help. A spokesperson for the society, as reported in the *Minneapolis Star Tribune*, said that implants account for a large chunk of surgeons' practices, including as much as 50 percent for some practitioners.[89]

Silicone Is Safe, Say Surgeons

"Silicone is used in practically everything," said Ronald Iverson, a California plastic surgeon and former chairman of the ASPRS's public education committee. "I think the people [speaking out against silicone implants] are a vocal minority."[90]

On January 19, 1992, shortly after the initial moratorium issued by FDA Commissioner Kessler, a team of Tampa-based plastic surgeons published an editorial in the *Tampa Tribune*—one of many across the United States—supporting this view: "We feel Kessler's decision is based on flawed and potentially fraudulent sources of information. We also feel he is under a great deal of pressure by special interest groups to remove breast implants from use for reasons not related to specific health factors regarding them."[91] These were strong words indeed—especially given the fact that the ASPRS was itself aggressively lobbying for continued use of implants. When presented with research about the dangers of implants, some plastic surgeons have been highly and openly skeptical. The *Wall Street Journal*, in a March 1992 article, reported that three men (including Frank Vasey) "suffered the same professional humiliation: When they warned plastic surgeons about possible problems with silicone breast implants, their warnings were rejected and they were condemned."[92] Plastic surgeons even began to assemble local panels to defend the safety of implants to the mass media as negative publicity broke. Said Tampa plastic surgeon William Luria: "A small group of people are doing a great deal of misleading. The studies are poorly written, poorly conceived . . . and filling up [medical] journals with garbage." [93]

If all the studies and opinions weren't valid, why didn't plastic surgeons themselves conduct research to check possible health risks? Did they simply accept everything the manufacturers told them? The practice of independent clinical testing of products takes place almost religiously in all fields of medicine with virtually all drugs and devices.

Five factors appear to have contributed to making the "silicone safety case" airtight in many surgeons' minds:

- Few problems were called to the attention of plastic surgeons by implant manufacturers.

- Few medical papers were published on silicone-induced complications and autoimmune conditions in plastic surgery peer-reviewed medical journals.

- Lack of regulatory pressure from the FDA left open the need for specific safety data.

- Thousands of surgeons were eager not to rock the political boat and so did not pay serious attention to the negative reports around them about silicone.

- There was an influx of positive, short-term feedback from implant recipients, which assured patient satisfaction for a job well done.

But as events implicating silicone gel with autoimmune and rheumatic illness unfolded, some patients interviewed and treated at the USF Division of Rheumatology contended that plastic surgeons in private practice took on a blame-everybody-but-me attitude. Admittedly, many plastic surgeons were not fully informed by either manufacturers or the FDA about some of the emerging issues, as we have already seen. In preparing this book, we extended an invitation to the ASPRS to state its views and position, but the organization, though polite (a nonmedical staff member returned our call), was unable to arrange a timely interview with an appropriate ASPRS surgeon spokesperson.

What Plastic Surgeons Were Told About Silicone Implants

Caveat emptor—"let the buyer beware"—was perhaps the unspoken cornerstone of manufacturers' marketing programs regarding breast implants. Interviews we have conducted suggest that on many occasions little information was given by implant sales representatives to surgeons about the lack of relevant immune-system clinical tests and many other possible side-effect risk factors. Both believed—or wanted to believe or were led to believe—that these products were safe, inert, and biocompatible.

In every field of medicine, manufacturers work hard to make claims for product efficacy and safety that neither invite disapproval from the FDA nor arouse the suspicions of physicians by exaggerating product performance. Most medical firms will push their claims to the limit, but not beyond. Additionally, all devote money—some more, some less—to advertising and promotion, and use the scientific studies and clinical experiences available to them to back up their marketing pitch and product positioning to the FDA, doctors, and consumers, as well as the medical and lay press. Sometimes the science is valid and on target; sometimes it's not. That's when some companies may start to fudge certain marketing claims, and that's why the FDA has recently made an effort to clamp down on companies who make claims for a product that are not in line with the strict usage and approval granted for it by the agency. In this regard, the implant industry has had a field day, since it remained virtually unregulated and unexamined for nearly three decades.

(The FDA has also acted in recent years to regulate more strictly manufacturers' practices of using paid consultants as "hired guns" to speak on their behalf at medical conferences, as well as to promote their products in a nonbalanced, biased manner. Today, such activities increasingly leave physicians, corporations, and their consultants open to the possibility of direct and costly judicial actions.)

Over the years, manufacturers and plastic surgeons relied heavily on each other for feedback on product performance, but they didn't always share information. No news was treated as good news by both parties, when it turned out to be very bad news for many women. At the same time, many of the issues that *were* acknowledged, such as the gel-bleed phenomenon, were treated as inconsequential; silicone was still thought to be inert.

The result? The implant business became very profitable for years-- until it was halted in early 1992. Though thousands of plastic surgeons claimed otherwise, a March 1992 *Wall Street Journal* article noted:

> There is evidence that over the past two decades . . . plastic surgeons themselves saw and ignored red flags in this lucrative branch of their specialty. Critics say many plastic surgeons failed to alert women to possible health risks reported by several sources, including professional journals, manufacturers and some of their own patients.
>
> This newspaper sent a reporter to four randomly chosen plastic surgery offices in New York City presenting herself as a candidate for surgery . . . [A]ll four [surgeons] recommended saline implants [yet] none mentioned the FDA's warnings that saline implants with silicone exteriors may . . . pose an increased risk of cancer and autoimmune disorders.[94]

Some plastic surgeons saw no problem at all; some looked the other way as the evidence mounted; some sensed what was happening but failed to address the medical issues and help solve the problem; and/ or some were left in the dark in areas in which they should have been better informed and more involved in information-gathering and problem-solving. Thousands of women patients claim that their plastic surgeons could and should have done more. Positive short-term patient results; peer pressure/group think and defensive ASPRS lobbying; the desire for ongoing financial success; a lack of scientific rigor, awareness, or openness to verifying outside medical research and issues; and a lack of orientation to internal medicine and clinical diagnoses—all of these factors influenced plastic surgeons and exacerbated the silicone implant problem for many years.

Some surgeons have stated that other technical issues served to complicate matters as well. Throughout the manufacturing history of implants, for example, various refinements were regularly made to the gel, specifically to its texture. The thickness of the outer jacket was also modified several times. As women presented problems to their plastic surgeons, many doctors simply replaced the original implants with an updated version—as often as four or more times in a single patient.

Both doctor and patient most likely assumed that some or all of the individual's problems resulted from an inferior implant, and that such problems would be resolved once new devices were in place. Did the repeated implantations take the surgeons' attention away from the true culprit—the elemental silicon and/or the silicone polymer in the gel and the particle-shedding envelope?

On the other side of the culpability coin, from 1982 to 1988, when the FDA finally began to get tough from a regulatory standpoint (though this movement was blunted to a certain degree by strong lobbying efforts by plastic surgeons on the FDA's medical-device advisory panel), about 500,000 women received silicone breast implants.[95] It's our opinion that during this time plastic surgeons were lax in their reporting of implant problems to the FDA.

Injection Procedure Defies FDA Mandate

A small number of plastic surgeons were also cited with having simply ignored the FDA's warnings about injectable silicone, even though these warnings were backed by significant evidence of the risk associated with these procedures. Documented medical effects of silicone injection have included everything from permanent sores and lumps to migration of silicone to the lungs, resulting in death. Injection of liquid silicone was made illegal back in 1965, except for doctors who obtained permits to conduct human experiments. Yet some doctors continued the practice without permits until June 1991, when the FDA commissioner issued a stringent warning that these injections were against the law. Currently, no doctor has authority for any experimentation.

Surgeons Demand Proof
to Legitimize Implant Moratorium

Plastic surgeons willingly agreed to comply with the FDA's moratorium on silicone-gel breast implants in January 1992, though most openly shared the opinion that the health risks of implants were being misrepresented and greatly exaggerated. According to a *New York Times* article, Norman Cole, former ASPRS president, said the moratorium had "created hysteria, anxiety and panic." He reportedly criticized FDA Commissioner Kessler for holding back scientific or medical information that would be useful to surgeons in making their own evaluation. Without access to this data, claimed Cole—the withholding of which was "unconscionable, an outrage"—the 3,850 certified plastic surgeons in the ASPRS were not equipped to offer medical opinions to frustrated implant patients who came to see them.[96]

Kessler countered Cole's assertion by noting that the information, which was subject to a federal court order preventing its dissemination, had raised unacceptable safety concerns. Many of the documents revealing important evidence had been sealed as a result of rulings in lawsuits against manufacturers. This lack of access to relevant data had delayed assessment by the FDA and its committees.

Questioning the Risk Data

Implants pose only a modest risk of capsular contracture, according to the ASPRS, which has maintained in its literature that this risk factor occurs in only 10 percent of women, while causing significant discomfort or alteration of shape in only the most severe cases. However, other data indicate that the frequency of contracture may be more than the ASPRS suggests—affecting 32 percent of USF patients. Making the issue still more unclear, one implant manufacturer, McGhan Medical Corporation, has said that capsular contracture can occur in as many as *74 percent* of patients. Whom should we believe?

Rupture risk has also been downplayed by some doctors. According to an article in *New Woman*, one patient was initially told by her plastic surgeon that "you could jump off the Empire State Building, and you'd be dead, but the implants would be intact." Two years later, the same surgeon told her (following implant rupture) that she was "the first woman in history ever to have this problem."[97] The year was 1986—24 years after the first silicone-gel implant. Why were there not more reports published in peer-reviewed plastic surgery literature from surgeons about implant rupture cases, and why wasn't more attention paid to what was published? Like the information concerning the risk of capsular contracture, the data on the risk of implant rupture is inconsistent and widely variable. Most women with implants told the authors they were advised by their plastic surgeons that the implants they received would last the rest of their lives. In the June 1992 *New England Journal of Medicine*, however, Jack Fisher, M.D., a plastic surgeon from the University of California in San Diego, noted a 4 to 6 percent rupture rate (although the findings did not indicate over what length of time these ruptures occurred). Hollis Caffee, M.D., a plastic surgeon at the University of Florida, Gainesville, noted in April of 1992 at the Public Health Service Implant Task Force that implants removed today which were made more than 10 years ago are almost always broken. Currently, an increasing number of physicians appear to believe that if an implant becomes ruptured, it should be removed.

Other risks not readily discussed were the possibility of complete loss of sensation in the breasts and the overall discomfort that might linger for months postoperatively. As for the information provided on product inserts, as of July 1992, only doctors practicing in Maryland were required to pass on any such information to their patients. It is our opinion that other educational pamphlets, even those from the FDA discussing infection, connective tissue disease, autoimmune disorders, and other medical problems, rarely found their way into patients' hands. (Today, many plastic surgeons provide implant patients with lengthy disclosures about potential complications.)

A 1991 ASPRS pamphlet entitled "Straight Talk About Breast Implants" (now out of print) stated that "breast implants are among the safest surgically implanted devices in use today. For the vast majority of women, the implant will come to feel like part of their bodies, occasionally subject to their own special 'illnesses' and injuries." The statement is vague enough to make the implants seem benign. The pamphlet goes on to say that "there have been some very rare cases reported in the medical literature in which women with breast implants developed some rare forms of arthritis-like diseases. It is not known for sure if the diseases were triggered in any way by the implants, but their development was probably coincidental." Is this responsible patient education or irresponsible public relations?

Saline Implants

Some surgeons who have long recommended saline implants to their patients say that their colleagues wouldn't use them because they were problematic to work with. Saline implants must be individually filled by a surgeon trained to do so, whereas silicone-gel implants come from the manufacturer ready for insertion. Even after it became clear that saline implants posed fewer risks—although they are not risk-free by any means—and after newer saline models reduced the risk of sudden deflation common in earlier versions, many surgeons were still not keen to use them.

Autoimmune and Rheumatic Disorders

"Whistleblowing" rheumatologists have been accused by many plastic surgeon groups of everything from poor diagnostic practices to unethical solicitation of patients to shamelessly seeking publicity for their findings about silicone disease.

The rheumatologist has thus often been cast, and openly attacked, as a doomsayer who has needlessly frightened women, while raking in large sums as an expert witness in lawsuits and closely guarding his scientific findings against objective evaluation. Yet most plastic surgeons have ignored their patients as a source of information. How can it be that the majority of women with the common constellation of symptoms in silicone-associated connective tissue disease show improvement following implant removal? Can this be dismissed as coincidental in case after case?

Even physicians from the surgeons' own camp have concurred that explantation often leads to improvement. Lu-Jean Feng, Clinical Assistant Professor of Surgery at Case Western University and a plastic surgeon in private practice in Cleveland, has spoken loud and clear about silicone-induced disease. "I think a silicone-associated illness exists in a susceptible group of the population," said Dr. Feng, in an interview. "I have found, first, that a lot of the patient's improvement following explantation is psychological. Additionally, I've found a greater than 90 percent improvement in the area of local symptoms: a reduction in pain as a result of scar tissue formation or inflammation in the breast and chest wall area. Regarding systemic symptoms—such as fatigue—I've personally found that about 33 percent of patients improve from six to twelve months following implant removal."

Feng has taken a lot of heat from her colleagues for her beliefs. "I don't feel good about what has been said about me by some, but this is the lot that I have to live with. I've taken on a controversial standpoint; this kind of viewpoint has tremendous effect on others' practice. But I believe things will get better as we learn more about the issues."

And Karen Wells, a plastic surgeon and Assistant Professor of Surgery at the University of South Florida Department of Plastic Surgery, has independently reported at a conference at H. L. Moffitt Cancer Center at the University of South Florida that 58 percent of her implant patients with rheumatic problems have shown improvement eight months after explantation. "I am impressed that some of my patients are quite ill, with no obvious *non-silicone* explanation," said Dr. Wells. "Some women who are asymptomatic are beginning to request implant removal as well."

An October 1992 article in *USA Today* quoted William W. Shaw, Professor and Chief, Division of Plastic Surgery, UCLA Medical Center, as finding that of the 150 patients from whom he removed breast implants, 90 percent obtained relief in localized pain such as burning of the chest wall, and 70 percent achieved systemic improvements for fatigue and for joint, muscle, and headache pain.[98] "This doesn't prove that implants cause immune problems," Shaw said, "because a placebo effect could at least partially explain why the symptoms improve. But it's my personal opinion that some of these women are very legitimate, and their symptoms are real."

There have been other recent studies, however, that show different silicone-associated connective tissue disease findings. At the October 1992 American College of Rheumatology meeting, three papers were presented that found no statistically significant difference regarding the onset of three specific rheumatic diseases in women with silicone implants and the general population. Fred M. Wigley, Clinical Director, Division of Rheumatology, Johns Hopkins School of Medicine, reported no difference in the frequency of scleroderma in silicone implant recipients versus the nonimplant population.[99] The study included 741 patients from Baltimore and Pittsburgh. In a separate study, Carin Dugowson, Assistant Professor of Medicine, Rheumatology, of the University of Washington in Seattle, noted that of 1,444 women who came to a breast cancer screening, less than 1 percent had breast implants.[100] They then looked at 299 women with recent onset of rheumatoid arthritis, finding that only one patient had implants. Thus, no differences were seen statistically between the two groups. And, finally, in a study funded by Dow Corning, John Goldman, a rheumatologist in private practice in Atlanta, found that in 99 implant patients monitored since 1985, 9 were found to have developed either rheumatoid arthritis or lupus, a percentage of illness onset matched in a control population.[101]

However, the majority of the other twenty papers presented at the rheumatology meeting did note connections between breast implants and immune dysfunction. More research is nevertheless needed in many areas. One good example of research progress is the way in which recent efforts have addressed concerns raised earlier by Noel R. Rose, Department of Immunology and Infectious Diseases, Johns Hopkins School of Hygiene and Public Health. Rose had commented that, in order to "show silicone is an antigen, one needs to demonstrate either silicone-specific antibodies or silicone-specific T cells. Thus far, neither of these demonstrations has been accomplished." This is important, Rose believed, so that a more definitive understanding of the possible connection between silicone breast implants and diseases having immunologic manifestations could be made. One of Rose's requirements has since been met by P. Heggers and his associates from the University of Texas at Galveston, who demonstrated antibodies to silicone in a work recently published in *Lancet*.[102]

On numerous occasions, plastic surgeons have not merely rejected but condemned the research of other medical professionals—and even manufacturers—who have mentioned the possibility of silicone-associated autoimmune disease in implant patients.

Consider, for example, the case of James Rudy, former president of the company which manufactured polyurethane foam–coated implants. When he urged doctors in 1976 to tell their patients about possible complications with these implants, he was told that he had "his head up his behind," according to an article in the *Wall Street Journal*.[103] That year, he sent a letter to surgeons requesting more data on how the implants had ruptured and how they had been implanted before breaking, but the letter generated very little interest.

A group of plastic surgeons also scoffed initially, said Melvin Silverstein, an oncologist, in the same *Wall Street Journal* article, when he told them in 1986 that silicone implants made mammograms hard to read. The surgeons reacted to his presentation by telling him to go study the issue again.[104] He has repeatedly confirmed his findings, which are now winning acceptance from plastic surgeons.

Toward Cooperation and a Solution

Did surgeons ineffectively educate their patients about risks? While it can be claimed that not enough information was made available to them to warrant such warnings to patients, it can also be claimed that they didn't keep their eyes and ears open to the emerging trends in the medical literature, nor did they actively pursue rigorous testing on their own. Regardless of manufacturers' lack of adverse-reaction data, many women presented surgeons with symptoms that didn't seem to add up. Moreover, the FDA had given a preliminary, and later an official, Class III designation to the devices: safety was unproven. And, finally, ASPRS pro-silicone-safety lobbying dollars were used to finance efforts to blunt negative implant publicity.

The time has come to work together to address this health care issue, because many women are sick and many more may become sick. For the medical profession to be at odds with itself is no answer to the call of the Hippocratic oath.

Part III:
You and Your Implants

Chapter 6

What You Should Do
About Your Implants

There were many, many nights I'd go to bed and not know if I was going to wake up in the morning . . . .

Katie decided to have implants when she was 27. Within a year, she started having trouble with capsular contracture on one of them, and went back to her surgeon for help.

"I had a closed capsulotomy [a nonsurgical manipulation to break up fibrous tissue to soften the breast] done manually in his office. My plastic surgeon told me it was no big deal," Katie explained. "I had both of my kids with me when I went, that's how easy I thought it would be. At the time, I didn't know that breaking the capsule was a no-no; nobody told me. After the procedure—he popped the hardened tissue in my breasts by hand without any anesthesia at all—I got back in my van and started to drive home. The next thing I knew, I totally blacked out on the highway—that's how bad the pain got. That doctors do this procedure to a human being without any anesthesia is unbelievable."

By the second year, Katie had developed a lump on the same breast near the nipple. Six months later, she began to feel chronically sick, and missed five straight weeks of work. Her abdominal pains got so bad that she underwent a laparoscopy. "They went through my belly button to look around," Katie said, "but they couldn't find anything wrong. Yet I was constantly running a fever from 99.5° to 102°, which never went back to normal until after I had the implants removed."

Katie had been working 60 hours a week as a credit manager, but had to cut back to under 20 hours due to her health. She got fired. She had no disability insurance to fall back on. "During this period, I saw 13 different doctors, and they all thought I had cancer—maybe lymphoma, maybe leukemia—or some infectious disease. I also had a chronic bladder infection. The doctors put me through every test imaginable. My white count went up to 22,000, even after five weeks of antibiotic therapy. My neck was very swollen on my left side. I was so sick I could hardly get out of bed. I was dying; there's no doubt in my mind I would have been dead had those things not been removed."

Finally, an oncologist noticed that she had vacuolated lymphocytes (white blood cells containing abnormal clear spaces) and suggested that she have the silicone implants removed. "Look, I don't believe it's my implants," Katie remembered telling the cancer specialist. "I didn't want it to be my implants. I loved my implants," she said.

After becoming increasingly ill, Katie finally did have them removed. Following the explantation, the surgeons informed her that "there was no doubt in their minds it was from the silicone," she said. "Then, after all I went through—my breasts are still completely numb—I finally went over the edge. I ended up in a mental hospital for two weeks. I'm on antidepressants, but I'm getting there. There are still some bad days, but they're a whole lot better.

"Now I wake up in the morning and think to myself, 'Thank God I'm alive,' instead of 'Oh, God, another day.' "

"The doctor told me my implants would never cause me problems." . . . "Maybe I'm just working too hard, or getting older." . . . "My husband loves the way my breasts look." . . . "I'd rather die than give up my implants . . . ."

For a wide variety of reasons, many women initially find it extremely difficult to accept that their chronic flulike symptoms, swollen glands, exhaustion, and other problems may be caused by silicone from their breast implants. That's because the cosmetic and psychological effects of this prosthetic device are powerful, especially in the first few years after implantation. Many women virtually "forget" they even have implants, thinking them as natural as their hands and feet.

For some, it is this psychological denial that is the single most difficult issue to overcome when they first become ill. Complicating matters is the fact that many plastic surgeons have repeatedly told their patients that implants couldn't possibly cause health problems. Accepting the possibility that *implants can be hazardous to your health* is the first step a woman experiencing rheumatic or autoimmune symptoms must take. She must allow herself to question the safety of the implants in her own body. And while this may sound obvious, it isn't: self-denial can be a very powerful thing.

"I didn't want it to be my implants," said Katie. "I loved my implants. I really did my homework before I got them, too. I got the opinion of two medical doctors. I got all the literature from the American Society of Plastic and Reconstructive Surgeons. My plastic surgeon even told me I'd be the firmest lady in my neighborhood when I was 65. Well, I'd like to see *his* wife with these things when she's 65—or his daughter," she said angrily.

Once a woman can acknowledge that her implants may be responsible for her health problems, it's often a scary emotional plunge. But it's equally important not to panic, because even if symptoms are silicone-related, they will not get worse in a day or a week (except in the case of a known rupture, which requires immediate attention). Most symptoms build slowly. Quick action is vital, but don't overreact; take the time to rule out all nonsilicone-related issues and make medical decisions that are rational. Explantation surgery comes with its own share of dangers and postoperative traumas, both physical and psychological, and it needs to be approached with caution and wisdom.

Unexplained Symptoms Should Not Be Taken Lightly

When most of us experience obvious or serious medical problems, we see a doctor. Yet since initial symptoms of silicone-induced disease are rarely well defined, they may be seen as "not serious enough" to interfere with one's life. That can be a costly oversight—especially in the critical early stages of the disease. Very often, women with silicone disease proceed from day to day, explaining away their bodies' reactions for long periods of time. Especially in the early phases of feeling ill, the vast majority of implant patients don't want to believe the problem is connected to their prostheses. This makes denial both easy and dangerous. And since a woman's health may remain stable at this stage of silicone disease, it's possible to miss all the clues. Only when symptoms and illness progress to the serious stage, as silicone continues to enter into tissue and lymph, stimulating an ever-increasing assault by the "supercharged" immune system, do the manifestations of the disease become undeniable.

To draw an analogy out of Hollywood, this scenario is reminiscent of the Hitchcock classic *Notorious*. In this film, Ingrid Bergman plays a character being slowly poisoned by her husband, played by Claude Rains. Each night, he puts a small amount of poison in a glass of warm milk and gives it to her. Each day, she becomes a little sicker. A doctor comes to examine her, but is unable to pin down the problem, and she almost dies. Then, in classic golden-era Hollywood style, Cary Grant discovers the murder plot and comes to her rescue.

Unfortunately, real life is no movie; Cary Grant is not waiting off-camera. Women with implants may be "ingesting" a steady flow of silicone into their bodies every day. That's why every woman with breast implants--even those without symptoms—must be highly vigilant regarding her health, carefully observing the following guidelines to ensure the rapid identification of any potential problems:

1. Closely monitor yourself to see if you have any of the symptoms described in chapter 2.

2. Check your breasts regularly to see whether their shape, texture, or size is changing.

3. Do not ignore common symptoms such as fatigue and muscle pain that persist over time, even if they seem like minor problems. Seek medical care before they escalate.

4. Notify any doctors you see that you have implants, so that any possible connection between symptoms and implants can be investigated.

5. If suspicious symptoms develop, see a rheumatologist or other physician experienced in the diagnosis and treatment of women with silicone-related problems.

Examine Your Breasts Regularly and Carefully

In addition to having regular breast checkups performed by an ob/gyn, an internist, or other health professional trained in breast examination, you should examine your breasts yourself every month. You can then become familiar with how the breast tissue feels normally, so that you'll recognize changes quickly that may indicate rupture or an immune response.

- *If you menstruate*, examine your breasts two or three days after the end of the menstrual period, when they are least likely to be tender or swollen.

- *If you do not menstruate*, make sure to examine your breasts at the same time of each month.

Here is a simple, step-by-step way to perform a thorough breast examination at home:

1. Stand in front of the mirror and check for anything that looks unusual, such as changes in the shape, size, firmness, or appearance of your breasts, nipples, and areola complex.

2. Raise the right arm above the head and use the fingertips of your left hand to feel for any unusual lump, swelling, or mass under the skin of the right breast. Feel for any swelling of lymph node glands or development of lumps in the underarm.

3. Reverse this process for the left breast.

4. Repeat these procedures for both breasts while lying down. This step is important, since in a prone position the breast tissue flattens, making possible palpation that can catch problems missed while standing.

Be sure to pay attention to areas of pain, tenderness, or color changes in the chest area. Also, watch for any discharges or unusual sensation around the nipple. If you experience any of these signs, be sure to report them without delay to your physician.

Understand What Mammograms Can and Cannot Do

Naturally, all women (with and without implants) should get mammograms and sonograms at recommended intervals. If you have had breast cancer surgery, be sure to ask your physician whether mammograms are still necessary.

Always inform a radiologist or X-ray technician about your implants before an examination. Obscuring of breast tissue during conventional mammography makes cancer screening difficult. From 25 percent to 85 percent of the tissue is blocked by a silicone-shelled implant. Therefore, it is possible for an implant patient to have a mammogram that shows no trace of disease only to discover later that her breast cancer went undetected.

X-rays cannot pass through a breast implant without casting a shadow on the film, blocking the view of some breast tissue. Granuloma formation, resulting from cells that surround escaped silicone droplets to form lumps in breast tissue, may also make tumor detection more difficult. Conversely, but less well known, silicone gel in surrounding tissue—due to an unnoticed rupture, for example—can be picked up by a mammogram, only to be *wrongly diagnosed* as a tumor.

If you don't want your implants removed unless you're absolutely sure that silicone is leaking into your body, mammography can *sometimes* detect a "silent rupture"—that is, when an implant ruptures but there are no symptoms. However, mammography is *not* advisable on a regular basis for young women who still have their own breast tissue, because it exposes them to more radiation, itself a cancer risk factor.

Today, advanced radiological techniques involving extra X-ray pictures and a method called displacement, in which breast tissue is compressed while the implant is pressed against the chest, may be able to provide a more valid reading. Some radiologists believe better definition of breast tissue can be obtained by a xeromammogram. Because it uses more radiation and more expensive materials, however, relatively few machines are available. Ultrasound is also thought to be helpful in the hands of experienced radiologists. More recent adaptations have been made to magnetic resonance imaging (MRI) as well, in order to allow precise study of the implants, silicone particles, surrounding breast tissue, and regional lymph nodes. The cost is much greater than traditional mammograms, however.

Do Not Delay Seeking Treatment

Some concerns have also been raised that women who fear they may have breast cancer delay seeking treatment because of the recent FDA moratorium on silicone-gel implants. They are terrified of the prospect of losing their breasts and being unable to get a prosthesis to replace them. Others simply cannot bear facing the bad news. Out of sheer repression, symptoms may be completely discounted and ignored. Remember: saline implants (which may also stimulate silicone disease but are probably safer—though they too are being examined by the FDA) remain on the market. If breast cancer is suspected, do not under any conditions avoid medical treatment; you may be risking your life. Keep in mind, furthermore, that not all women with breast cancer require mastectomy. A lumpectomy—the removal of only the tumorous lump instead of the whole breast—is often performed instead, depending on the extent of the cancer and when it was diagnosed.

Removing or Keeping Silicone Implants: A Double-Edged Sword

Deciding whether to have your silicone-gel prostheses explanted can be an extremely tough choice. On the one hand, it should be clear they can, and do, harm susceptible women's health. On the other hand, plastic surgeons and many other physicians continue to say that there's no proven and legitimate reason to remove them, and that the connection between the immune system and silicone disease is purely coincidental, anecdotal, and hypothetical. Just look at the majority of implant recipients who are well, they say.

Besides, who would ever opt for more surgery? All surgical procedures are scary and at least somewhat risky, even under ideal conditions. If surgery can be reasonably avoided, it should be. Additionally, there is the nonreimbursable cost of explantation. Though some plastic surgeons have been reported to remove the prostheses from their own patients without charge, other surgeons have charged from $1,500 to as much as $30,000—in cases where leaked silicone gel needs to be removed from large areas of the chest.

The following is a discussion of the major issues that cause many women considering implant removal to vacillate, plus some advice on what action might make things a bit easier.

1. Risks of Surgery

Any additional surgery puts an implant recipient at risk. The complications that follow cutting into the skin and manipulating the soft tissues of the chest include the possibility of local or systemic infection; reactions to anesthesia; additional scarring; and drooping breast tissue.

Also, scarring from the original implant procedure will, in most cases, have had a detrimental effect on blood supply to that area of the breast. This can increase the likelihood of surgical complications, including *hematoma* (bleeding from a ruptured blood vessel), following secondary surgical procedures such as explantation.

Some surgeons have begun to use lasers and electrocauterization to stop bleeding as part of the overall explantation procedure. Just as laser surgery has greatly decreased the trauma and recovery time of a wide range of surgeries (due to reduced invasion of, and trauma inflicted upon, the body), the use of advanced technologies like these may help to limit possible surgical difficulties. Lasers may be unwise, however, in removing polyurethane-coated implants because of the concern regarding possible tolulene production.

2. Disfigurement

In some women, the cosmetic results of implant removal have been poor, since any breast tissue that remains runs the risk of atrophy due to implantation and exposure to surgical trauma. This may lead to a varying and unpredictable degree of disfigurement, along with smaller breasts because of the tissue and muscle loss.

It is also important to realize that a surgeon cannot know to what degree the silicone-gel implant's jacket has been "eaten" by immune system macrophages, or how much scar tissue or gel is in the body until he or she sees it during the actual operation. Thus, it is difficult to gauge in advance how much tissue will need removal. Again, mammograms cannot offer any reliable advance warning, either. If the gel has entered the pectoral (chest) muscles, the surgeon may have to remove some tissue in an effort to clear away immune-system-triggering silicone; this can cause chest *concavity* in the breast area. More scarring is also likely, based on how much natural breast tissue remains, as well as on the range of inflammation caused by the silicone particles surrounding the implant.

Some women opt for saline-filled implants to replace the gel-filled prostheses. That is a personal decision based on the degree of risk one is willing to live with. Other women choose to get no replacement. Yet another possibility is a TRAM (transverse rectus abdominis myocutaneous) flap procedure. Here, a woman's skin, fat, and underlying muscle are surgically transferred—while remaining connected to the original blood supply from the abdomen—to rebuild the breast without an implant. Postoperatively, a nipple-areola complex is then literally tattooed in place to create the impression of a replacement. Very thin women are not candidates, as some bulk is needed to perform this surgery successfully. The overweight get an added advantage: a tummy tuck.

The other side of the TRAM flap coin is that complications can include breast tissue that dies due to failed blood supply—a problem in up to 10 percent of cases. The surgery is also long: five to seven hours.

Other women have been able to have their breasts reshaped with autologous fat transplantation. This technique "borrows" portions of the body's fat from areas with extra amounts and moves it into the breast. Since this tissue is one's own, there's no risk of rejection or immune response. Unfortunately, this process has several drawbacks, according to plastic surgeons: not all the fat injected will survive, and when it dies it can cause little calcium specks that cannot be distinguished from cancer specks on a mammogram. It is also very costly—about $10,000 per breast—and time-consuming for both surgeon and patient. Not all women can have one, either, due to various patient selection criteria. The procedure also requires a subsequent procedure to reconstruct the nipple-areola complex.

Please see Appendix A for other alternatives and a complete discussion.

3. Greater Loss of Sensitivity

Secondary surgical procedures such as explantation have been known to cause further loss of sensitivity in the breasts and nipples due to additional nerve damage and blood flow restrictions, exacerbating numbness noted by patients following their original surgery.

A woman considering implant removal should speak honestly with her surgeon to discuss how the surgery will be done—and how much risk it will involve of further sensitivity loss.

4. No Guarantee of Postoperative Improvement

In research conducted at USF and elsewhere, implant removal has led to symptomatic improvement in approximately 70 percent of patients in an average of two years after removal. Some women get completely better; others get a little or a lot better, but do not recover completely. In other cases, a blunting of further medical deterioration is achieved, but symptoms do not improve. And in a small number of women, conditions continue to worsen even after implant removal, due to a concurrent, nonsilicone-related rheumatic condition; an immune system irreversibly affected by silicone before explantation; or the continued stimulation of the immune system by silicone gel not fully retrieved from the body.

It should be underscored that many patients have been badly affected by leaked gel which could not be cleared surgically from tissues and the lymphatic system. Surgeons can locate gel only by eye, and even with the use of a high-powered surgical microscope, it is impossible to detect tiny particles that have ensconced themselves in tissue and migrated throughout the lymphatic system and various organs.

On a more positive post-op recovery note, some patients taking drugs such as cortisone for treatment of silicone-related connective tissue disease may be able to stop this medication after explantation. (Since cortisone is a powerful medication, it often causes many negative side effects, especially when taken over a long period of time.)

5. Loss of Positive Self-image

It is no secret that women's self-image and body image are deeply entangled. Blame it on men, TV, the movies, advertising, *Penthouse* and *Playboy* magazines—it makes no difference. Women have internalized the beauty mandate, and many have come to accept it. At USF, one woman openly admitted that she would rather kill herself than have her breast implants out, no matter how terrible she might feel (she later changed her mind). Women who turned to silicone implants to solve their body- and breast-image concerns through augmentation simply cannot bear the feeling of "once again being ugly," "defective," "physically inadequate," "deformed"—among scores of other painful adjectives we have heard. The thought of removal is even worse for women who received their implants following mastectomy—these women would lose their breasts *twice*.

Obviously, cosmetic and psychological concerns must be balanced against physical and medical well-being. What are looks worth? How important is feeling well? How will the overall quality of life be improved by the removal? How will the loss of implants affect sex life, relationship, even career (for performers or models, for example). Remember: *symptoms may worsen if implants are not removed*, but guarantee for some degree of recovery is realistically 70 percent—not

100 percent. Your best bet is to talk with other women in similar situations. Get a lot of feedback from professionals, too: surgeons, physicians, a psychologist whom you trust. It is a deeply personal decision that no one can make for you.

6. Your Symptoms May Not Be Caused by Silicone

Silicone disease *mimics* certain rheumatic conditions, and it is possible that your health problems are not, either in whole or in part, due exclusively to the silicone-gel implants. Explantation is always a gamble to one degree or another, yet a solid clinical diagnosis of silicone-associated connective tissue disease, based on the previously described constellation of symptoms, will serve to point the patient firmly in the right direction. However, having the implants removed—along with all the trauma of surgery and postoperative physical and emotional recovery—may not resolve the medical problems.

The key here is to work closely with a qualified physician capable of noting subtle differences between silicone-related and typical rheumatic conditions. Along with the recognition that differentiation is difficult, you should also take advantage of resources that will enable you to contact other women who can share your knowledge and experiences. (See Appendix B for a current listing.)

7. Resistance from Your Surgeon

Some plastic surgeons have been noted by patients to refuse to remove implants even when the patient has pleaded for explantation; they deny that the implants have anything to do with the illness, or they do not want any further entanglement in the patient's problems. Luckily, as the evidence against silicone grows, more surgeons are treating requests for explantation seriously. The legal implications are also having a clear effect on surgeons' attitudes.

Ask your plastic surgeon to call your rheumatologist or physician for a medical discussion about your problem. If your surgeon still resists your request, find another surgeon who will remove your implants without giving you a hassle.

8. Reaction of a Mate

In our experience at USF, most patients' husbands or partners concur with the decision to have the implants removed. While we've come across cases in which a husband has been confused and unsupportive of his wife's medical condition in the early phase of silicone disease, we've yet to see a man encourage his spouse to keep her implants just because they enhance her physical attractiveness. Most husbands are far more concerned about what can be done to increase their wives' energy level and health than their bustlines.

A small number of women, especially those married long after getting implants, have never told their partners about their breast augmentation. The scars may be hard to see, and the husband (for one reason or another) never finds out. Obviously, this situation makes it more difficult to broach the subject of removal. A marriage counselor or therapist may be helpful in a situation when an objective, professional third party is needed to open up communication and feelings.

Of course, assuming the relationship can handle it—and a small minority cannot, by the way—it's a good idea to keep your partner fully apprised of your health condition and history. Not only will this allow him to be more fully supportive and involved, it can also ease your feelings of isolation, fear, and depression. The more open talk about what silicone disease is all about, the better it is for the couple in terms of coping with illness, making difficult medical decisions, and dealing with explantation-related medical and emotional issues—from finances to sex.

If your partner cannot accept or deal with your illness or the loss of your implants, then he needs help himself. Sadly enough, relationships have been reported to end because of this issue. In this regard, once again, support groups can help: if you know other women who have the same problems, perhaps your husband could talk to their husbands. If all else fails, the decision between health and relationship must ultimately be made.

○ *I've lost all my vanity . . . .*

After a double mastectomy, Irene soon became seriously ill from her implants; it's been nearly five years since she's had them removed. Today, she has silicone granulomas in her liver and spleen, silica in her lungs, severe autoimmune insulin-dependent diabetes, and chronic fatigue, and she must use an electric scooter to get to church, visit her doctor, and do grocery shopping.

"When I was an insurance agent, I had twelve other agents under me, and I worked twelve hours a day, six or seven days a week," Irene said. "Now I don't have a life. I get up, eat breakfast, and go back to bed; then I take a shower, and go back to bed; then I eat lunch, and go back to bed. My life is completely nil. It's very traumatic to lose your breasts once, but when you lose them again . . . ," she trailed off.

Irene blames plastic surgeons for misleading women about implants by not providing real information. She blames the FDA for not doing anything about problems as they developed. "I feel we were used as guinea pigs, and I feel we're still being used that way," she explained.

"I also believe in my heart that surgeons know what's going on today, but they're all chicken—afraid of their peers, afraid of lawsuits. They just don't want to get involved."

After years of illness and pain, Irene says that her attitudes have changed drastically regarding the importance of beauty. "You have to be thin, attractive, do everything for the outside. I had large breasts. Men were very attracted to me. But I'm so different now. I see that if someone doesn't want me because of my physical appearance, they are not worth wanting," she said. "And while women's attitudes are changing, there are still women who haven't gotten sick enough to lose their vanity, haven't gotten to the point where they say it's the inside that counts."

9. Surgical Expense

Ironically, explantation generally costs more than implantation. Furthermore, insurance reimbursement is very uncommon because silicone disease remains an "unproven" illness. There have been reports by USF patients of employers not even granting sick days or leaves of absence for silicone disease problems.

If you break down your treatment into different components on your insurance claim forms, your policy may cover you for some of the costs. Discuss this option with your surgeon and physician, or speak to your insurance broker or employee benefits manager at work for help. Your physician must emphasize to the insurance company that you are removing the implants for medical—not cosmetic—reasons.

I was ashamed to go to the doctors, because they didn't think anything was wrong with me . . . .

Wendy got implants because she didn't have much of a bust, and her husband wanted her to improve her appearance. She soon developed chronic respiratory problems (the diagnosis was asthma) and received steroid shots every two to four weeks for seven years, to no avail. Her marriage eventually ended, she slowly lost her health completely from a range of rheumatic ailments, and she wound up so distraught that she tried to take her own life with codeine pills, Valium, and whisky.

After finally being diagnosed with silicone-associated connective tissue disease at USF, Wendy saw a plastic surgeon who told her that there was no relation between her implants and her problems. "The surgeon, a woman, told me I was going to be deformed and ugly, my chest would be sunken, and that I was going to be scarred," Wendy said. "I still wanted them out."

Wendy had to wait four months to have her implants removed after deciding to get rid of them, because the insurance company wouldn't cover the procedure until she presented letters from two other doctors.

After explantation, she requested to go on light duty at work for a while, but the company doctor told her there was no relation between her implants and her problems of joint pain and muscle pain. Then she was told that she would be fired unless she found another position in the company within 90 days. Luckily, her union protected her and she kept her job. Even better, her silicone-related symptoms have improved dramatically since she got rid of her implants. "My ears do not ring anymore. No more headaches, bouts of vomiting and diarrhea, bronchial spasms, or hair loss," she said.

When You Should Get Rid of Your Implants and When You Shouldn't

After learning about all the possible dangers of silicone-associated connective tissue disease, you may assume that all of the estimated 1 million women who have them should seriously consider removal as quickly as possible. But that's only one side of the picture. Here's the way to approach the issue reasonably:

- *If you do have signs and symptoms of silicone disease*, arrange to have your implants removed as soon as possible in a best attempt to alleviate your signs and symptoms, while keeping a clear view on the possible explantation risks.

  In most cases—7 out of 10—the sooner a woman with silicone-induced disease rids herself of the implants, the better the likelihood of full or partial recovery. While some patients opt to replace silicone with saline implants, this decision should be thought through carefully since these implants contain silicone and silica and may also lead to an immune response in susceptible individuals. (This, however, is a personal decision based on severity of illness and personal risk/appearance values.)

- *If you don't have symptoms of silicone disease*, you do not have to rush to have your implants removed. You may be one of the large and fortunate majority who never become ill. Still, it is critical that you monitor yourself carefully on a regular basis for any of the trouble indicators. If you believe you are beginning to note signs and symptoms, meet with your physician to rule out other disorders, then with your plastic surgeon to arrange removal if silicone disease is a serious concern.

  It is also important that you check for systemic rheumatic symptoms and silicone-related disease as long as you have your implants. Maintain a health diary and monitor any pain or symptoms, such as muscle and joint pain, that occur in the absence of physical activity; or chronic fatigue that cannot be traced to anything specific, like an infection. Keep up with new medical information. Also, be sure to know your implant manufacturer, brand name, and type in the event that information specific to your prostheses is published.

If I Feel Okay Now, Am I Still at Risk?

Regrettably, the answer is yes.

Silicone implants may cause chronic immune system stimulation. And while every woman with implants has a different risk probability—some are clearly higher than others—the amount of time and silicone needed to precipitate a susceptible individual's silicone disease onset is not predictable. All we can be sure of is that the more silicone that gets into the body, the greater the risk of debilitating autoimmune/rheumatic disease.

Conclusion

The silicone breast implant controversy represents a massive failure of government, industry, and medicine to regulate and evaluate medical devices. It also exemplifies the risks posed to all Americans regarding the effects of poor communication, inexcusable indifference, and lack of cooperation. In short, the FDA, physicians, and industry failed to study and address properly the problems induced by the implantation of silicone implants into the bodies of an estimated 1 million women in the United States.

Many lessons must be learned in order to prevent the recurrence of any such future medical disasters. The Food and Drug Administration needs to develop new regulatory procedures aimed at evaluating medical devices with standards more closely in line with those of pharmaceutical products. Additionally, medical manufacturers and physician groups need to improve how they communicate concerning new and emerging health care problems; the overt expression of disagreement and hostility over issues must be replaced with team-work to solve problems.

Regarding the issue of medical disabilities from silicone disease, it must be acknowledged that women with this illness have a legitimate medical problem. Some have severe disability and cannot work. Government, insurance companies, and the health care profession need to face up to this reality and to address the issues of disability and medical reimbursement for treatment fairly.

For women, it would be a wonderful and positive step if attitudes could change regarding the ability to differentiate between idealistic "external" (societal) appearance and deeper, inner values of self-worth, knowing that breast size or bodily appearance is not the only—or most important—reflection of a person's beauty, talent, or value as a human being. Such thinking would quite dramatically impact the need for cosmetic breast augmentation in the first place.

Concurrently, for those women who are presently augmented—and for those who make the personal decision for augmentation in the future—there are many points which should be kept clearly in mind. First, it is often difficult for some women to accept that implants may be the cause of unexplained health problems, especially those who are otherwise pleased with their appearance. Accepting the possibility that implants can be hazardous to your health is often a critical first step toward diagnosis and recovery.

Additionally, patients should remember that a certain amount of silicone leaks, or bleeds, through the envelope of all silicone-gel implants, even in the absence of rupture. Thus, all women with silicone implants experience some exposure to the gel. Silicone particles shed from the outside of saline-filled envelopes as well. Again, women who have implants, and those considering them, need to realize that silicone-induced illness is unpredictable and may begin at any time. And while every woman with implants has a different risk probability, the great majority, in fact, may never be systemically affected by silicone, according to current medical opinion. What's more, the amount of time and silicone needed to precipitate any given individual's illness is not predictable.

Many of the illnesses reported by women with silicone breast implants are rheumatic in nature, affecting the body's joints, muscles, and connective tissues. Furthermore, a common constellation of symptoms shows up in a high percentage of women with implants who develop problems. While these specific symptoms also occur in the absence of breast implants, the more symptoms present in the absence of any obvious medical explanation, the more likely that silicone is the cause. However, not all women susceptible to silicone-associated connective tissue disease experience every symptom of the illness; the degree of severity varies widely according to each individual's duration and extent of exposure, as well as her genetic makeup and immune system.

The only currently available treatment is to rid the body of as much silicone as possible, primarily through surgical removal of the implants and the fibrous tissue around them. Because we lack specific cures, rheumatic disease treatment generally is based on the individual patient's symptom complex. Silicone patients are therefore managed in the same way as natural rheumatic disease patients. Symptomatic relief for some patients has been found in aspirin and aspirinlike medications called nonsteroidal anti-inflammatory drugs. In difficult circumstances, tricyclics like amitriptyline (used for central pain blocking and sedation), cortisone, hydroxychloroquine, and other immunosuppressive approaches may be tried.

In our initial experience based on the first 50 patients seen at USF, implant removal results in some degree of systemic improvement in approximately 70 percent of women within two years of explantation; improvement of localized symptoms has been reported to be even higher. In any case, it is critically important that any woman suspecting silicone illness seek medical treatment from the best possible health care provider. The right physician/illness "fit" must be made to ensure that the person receives optimal diagnosis and treatment. Doctors, on the other hand, generally need to improve how they work with their patients. Should an individual complain of a combination of symptoms not readily found in the medical literature, the physician ought not conclude by this fact alone that a person's condition is psychosomatic.

Patients sometimes lose faith in their doctors if problems cannot be readily resolved; at the same time, it is important to avoid blind faith in one's physician. People must realize that while the FDA, medical manufacturers, and physicians often do a good job regarding safety and patient protection, they cannot be relied on in every case. Patients need to take responsibility for their own health and health care, seeking to be as well educated as possible regarding the medical treatment they receive. If one has personal medical issues or questions that cannot be adequately addressed, the person should continue to seek help until a satisfactory level of understanding and care is obtained.

Above all, believe in yourself, and keep searching for answers that make you comfortable and address your needs.

Appendices

Appendix A

Implantation and Explantation Surgery

I wish I kept the cysts I had in my breasts, and I would be fine now . . . .

When Jane was 49, in 1974, her doctor recommended a subcutaneous mastectomy due to a recurring problem with multiple cysts in both breasts. The medical thinking at the time was that such a condition was likely precancerous (today it is approached less drastically, as the majority of these cysts are benign, though they do make breast cancer detection more difficult). The surgery was performed, and two silicone-gel implants were put in.

A few months after getting her implants, Jane began having severe chest pains, palpitations, and a fluctuation in her blood pressure. Soon she began experiencing arrhythmias and joint pain. Before long, she was suffering from capsular contracture in both breasts as well, and she had her implants replaced with saline-filled ones in 1976. Over the next three years, she developed worsening chest pains that moved down her arms, stomach and abdominal cramps, urinary tract infections, insomnia, and terrible headaches. Finally she fell into a deep depression requiring a psychiatrist's help. All the while EKGs, stress tests, barium enemas, angiograms, and other tests showed nothing. For a time, Jane's physician thought she might have a subdural hematoma in her brain, but that test turned out negative as well.

One of her new saline implants deflated in 1979 and the other one capsulated again, so she received implants a third time. Within a week, her breast area became red and began to look infected. A month later, one of the implants had begun to protrude through her skin. A serious staph infection set in, and Jane was hospitalized. She developed thrombophlebitis and vertigo, her headaches worsened, and she contracted a respiratory infection and later pneumonia—several times.

"Over the years, I have been on so many anti-inflammatory drugs and blood pressure medications, I've become allergic to them," said Jane, now 67. "I've been more than tortured. Last October, my husband had heart bypass surgery. I think all this finally caught up with him."

Today, over a year after having her implants removed for good, Jane can't even wear a bra because it hurts her chest too much. "And it's made a totally terrible thing out of our whole life as far as finances go . . . everything has gone down the drain."

The decision to have breast augmentation surgery calls into question a profound array of highly personal physical, psychological, and medical issues. So does the decision to undergo an explantation procedure due to silicone-induced illness or prosthesis injury, for example. Both types of breast surgery confront a woman with a wide range of possible ramifications, which can swing her life in a new direction.

We live in a world of medical miracles. Life expectancy and the quality of health care have reached new and unprecedented peaks and will continue to improve. Some of the biggest advances in medical care have occurred in the field of surgery: physical intervention within the human frame, capable, at its height of success, of restoring life and health when disease might otherwise have left the body permanently disabled or unable to function at all.

Having reached such a point of development, surgery has been able to move from resolving *needs*—as in "without the operation, the patient will die"—to addressing *wants*. Here we come upon the field of "elective" surgery, procedures not medically necessary but personally desirable. And for 8 in 10 breast implant recipients, looking and feeling better were their objectives; for the explant patient, feeling better is the single goal. Yet the means to both of these ends is *surgery*, a word with a connotation of danger, however "safe" an operation may be. This appendix examines the range of approaches a surgeon can take with breast implants, while addressing relevant surgical risk factors needed to complete the medical picture so that you can make the most informed decision possible regarding implantation or explantation.

Breast Augmentation Surgery: An Overview

Typically, women who consult a plastic surgeon to discuss breast augmentation are between 17 and 50 years of age. These women are often from one of two groups:

- Women who feel they have inadequate natural development of breast size or shape, or
- Women whose breasts have significantly changed to an undesirable appearance or size, most commonly following childbirth or weight loss.

Insurance rarely covers cosmetic augmentation; nor do many insurance carriers offer reimbursement for the treatment of medical problems during or after the surgical procedure itself. As noted, expenses for explantation are often not reimbursable either. Thus, all medical fees—for cosmetic implantation, complications, and explantation—are often borne directly by the patient.

Augmentation and explantation surgery may be performed in a hospital operating room, an outpatient ambulatory-care surgical center, or an accredited office surgery facility. Any emergency can occur during an operation, and the medical facility must be prepared for all possible contingencies. Personal recommendation from other patients is a common and helpful path to follow when searching for a surgeon and health care institution. (The ASPRS and local medical societies can also make recommendations for properly accredited and licensed health care providers.)

Each plastic surgeon takes a slightly different course of action regarding patient counsel and preoperative preparation for breast augmentation surgery. The following outline lists general areas of focus that should be covered.

1. Determination of patient motivation.

Most plastic surgeons will diligently confirm that the woman is well grounded regarding her personal decision to have implants. The surgeon will often conduct an interview to determine whether "exclusion criteria" are encountered, that is, whether a prospective patient is a poor implant candidate.

Such criteria might cover the case of a woman who wants breast enlargement following a rebound from a recent divorce or bereavement, or as a means of keeping a marriage together in the absence of counseling or other emotionally directed, problem-solving efforts. One surgeon mentioned an atypical, but frightening, case in which a woman requested implants for her daughter. "She doesn't go out with anyone because she's flat-chested, and she'd have a better chance of dating if she had better-developed breasts," the surgeon reported the mother as saying. (In such a case, the daughter would be asked her opinion privately.) In most cases, however, women seek breast augmentation as a means to feel better about themselves.

2. Evaluation of physical condition.

The woman should be given a thorough physical examination to determine general health as well as any contraindications for augmentation. A woman may be rejected for surgery should she have heart or lung disease, for example. Doctors may also advise against implants if there's a high genetic risk of breast cancer in her family, due to the possible obstruction of breast cancer screening techniques. Today, some plastic surgeons are advising women with *preexisting* lupus, scleroderma, rheumatoid arthritis, or other autoimmune disorders to be examined and cleared for surgery first by a rheumatologist or other physician able to evaluate autoimmune risk factors for a given individual. We believe these patients should not have implants placed.

3. Description of surgical risk factors.

There are many possible risks directly related to breast surgery itself. The following are some of the major areas to be aware of.

A. Infection

All surgical procedures involve risks to patients. The trauma of surgery lowers a patient's resistance to potentially dangerous local or systemic infection, which may result in serious illness following the operation. Such infection, while infrequent, usually occurs within a few days post-op. A fever of 101° or greater is a danger sign.

Women who develop infections that do not respond to medication must have their implants removed. If removal is required, the patient will have to wait between six weeks and six months after the infection has cleared before reinsertion of another implant is possible, if so desired.

B. Inflammation

Swelling or inflammation surrounding the breast area where surgery is performed is a normal occurrence; it is the body's way of reacting to injury. The time it takes for inflammation to subside varies according to the nature of the surgery and the overall health of the individual. Severe and sudden swelling and redness, however, which may occur on one side only, is not normal and should be reported immediately. Firmness in either or both breasts should also be watched for and reported.

C. Hematoma

A blood clot, called a hematoma, may form, due to blood vessel leakage; this may lead to discoloration, pain, localized inflammation, and swelling. There have also been reports of increased long-term risk of capsular contracture in patients who experience hematoma postoperatively.

D. Incision Drainage and Pain

A small amount of bloody drainage is normal and may occur at the incision site during the first postoperative day. However, more than a little drainage from the breast or the suture lines is not normal and requires immediate attention.

A mild to moderate degree of pain should also be expected. Pain and sleeping medications may be prescribed during this early phase. Severe, sudden onset of pain is a sign of problems, however.

E. Skin Necrosis

A blackening of breast skin tissue, called necrosis, is due to insufficient blood supply to the area. This can be caused by the skin being stretched too tightly over the implant, the result of an implant that is too large for the available tissue.

Since blood is required to deliver nutrients and remove waste products from all parts of the body, any damage to blood vessels within the breast during implantation (for example, hematoma) can result in the damage or death of healthy breast tissue. Also, since body fluids cannot travel freely through the implant, the device must be carefully situated to facilitate necessary, natural circulation.

Necrosis has also been reported due to radiation treatments, side effects from steroid medications used to treat capsule contracture, and smoking. In severe cases, the implant has been noted to come through the skin.

F. Reactions to Anesthesia

Patients should be informed of the pros and cons of general anesthesia (being put out completely), local anesthesia (localized numbing of the area), or a combination of local with mild sedation (being half asleep).

Some people react severely to anesthesia, suffering afterward from vomiting or more serious conditions. These responses are usually temporary. The anesthesiologist should also be notified of specific drugs that have caused problems in the past, so that substitutions can be made.

G. Other

Damage or nicks to the implant jacket upon implantation (with the saline implants available today, this will lead to deflation of the prosthesis).

- Asymmetry and/or improper placement of implants, which may leave the breasts unbalanced or misshapen, or may cause pain from pressure being placed against adjacent muscles and nerves. This condition can also negatively affect blood circulation.

- Capsule formation, which has been fully discussed earlier. It may be addressed via either a closed (not recommended) or open capsulotomy (an invasive surgical procedure posing other risk factors).

- Decreased sensation, which may be a complete or partial loss of sensation in the nipple, areola, or other areas of the breast as a result of damage to the nerves. This condition can lead to a change in sexual response.

- Oversensitization of the breast, nipple, or areola complex after surgery. This condition can also lead to a change in sexual response.

- Skin loss, which may result from atrophy of skin as a result of the trauma of surgery. There may also be a painful tightening of the skin around the breast.

- Scarring, which may be barely noticeable or apparent, depending on the woman's anatomy, the size of the implants, the type of incision, and the skill of the surgeon.

- Wrinkling of the implant, where visible folds in the implant jacket can be seen through the skin of the breast.

- Serious fluid accumulation around the implant following surgical placement. Aspiration, which poses numerous risks such as implant damage, may be used to reverse this problem. Persistent fluid accumulation necessitates prosthesis removal.

- The recovering patient will need to avoid reaching up or out for about three days; she should also sleep on her back with her head elevated for about seven days. Normal activities can usually be resumed gradually after one week's time, with more strenuous activities avoided for approximately three weeks post-op.

4. Discussion of incision options.

Although the surgeon will make a recommendation, the type of incision used is most often selected by the patient. There are three standard types used in implantation (recovery time is similar for all three, and each has its own pros and cons):

A. Inframammary incision
Probably the most commonly used incision, it is made under the breast at the fold or crease line. Its most significant disadvantage: the scar may be visible when a bra or bikini top is worn. This incision is typically about 2 inches in length.

B. Axillary incision
This incision is made in the axilla, or armpit. It is used less frequently due to the difficulty of properly placing the implant in some patients. Another disadvantage is that, in the event of a problem with the implant itself, an incision is often needed on the breast to gain access to the prosthesis.

C. Periareolar incision
Made around the nipple and areola complex, this incision has the drawback in some women of being too small to allow insertion of the implant.

5. Discussion of implant and implant placement.

The surgeon should discuss the two brands of implants available today, McGhan and Mentor. Both offer only saline-filled devices with a silicone jacket, either smooth or textured. The textured jacket is reported to lessen the possibility of capsular contracture. (It is hypothesized, however, that the increase of surface area to the immune system with a textured implant may actually increase the likelihood of capsule formation. Long-term studies are required.)

Regarding the selection of an implantation site, there are two possible locations:

A. Subglandular or submammary

This location rests between the breast tissue and the muscles of the chest wall. It is the most favored site, since situating the implant here is easiest to accomplish and usually results in less postoperative pain. It is also recommended for women with some, but not excessive, breast ptosis (sagging) to offer a degree of uplifting of the breast. Disadvantage: a subglandular implant may be more noticeable in slender women and has been noted to interfere more with mammography.

B. Submuscular

Situated between the muscles of the chest wall and the rib cage, this placement results in a more attractive breast, especially for slender women. Disadvantage: more pain after surgery, and certain muscle actions will cause the breast to move.

Implantation surgery generally takes from 45 minutes to 2 hours, depending on the surgeon and the specifics of the case. Incisions are closed with stitches, and a tape and dressing may be applied. Stitches are removed within five to seven days.

It is recommended that the patient be seen by the surgeon the day after surgery, at three days post-op, weekly for the first month, and at three-month intervals for the first year. Women should be seen by the surgeons annually thereafter and, of course, by their regular physicians on a routine basis.

Reconstruction

Women who want implants for breast reconstruction present an entirely different psychological and medical profile than those seeking cosmetic enhancement. For one thing, they face greater risks if recently recovering from cancer; their breasts and entire body have already been traumatized by radical surgery. Additionally, reconstructive surgery, done under general anesthesia, is lengthy—from two to seven hours in most cases. Insurance reimbursement for implantation for reconstructive purposes is customary, however.

Two additional steps are needed for reconstructive surgery:

1. Tissue expansion.

Depending on how much skin and breast tissue has to be removed, a new space for placing the implant may have to be created underneath the skin. The space is created by using a tissue expander, a temporary implant shaped like a breast prosthesis that is placed underneath the skin and muscle—either immediately after the breast is removed or a few weeks later—and is periodically inflated with saline solution. The amount of solution is increased gradually to enhance the shape. Once the skin has been sufficiently expanded, a permanent implant is inserted into the space.

2. Rebuilding the nipple-areola complex.

This part of the breast is created in a separate procedure after implantation. It is accomplished with plastic surgery dyes, in a process somewhat similar to tattooing.

Plastic surgeons may also employ other means of rebuilding the breast. The first, discussed previously, is called a TRAM flap procedure. The surgeon may also utilize a procedure known as a local muscle flap, in which a muscle is moved from the back, swinging tissue forward. This is similar to a musculocutaneous flap, in which both skin and muscle are moved from the back to rebuild the breast. There is also a procedure called a free flap, which involves taking a part of the buttock muscle, along with artery and vein, in order to rebuild the breast.

Explantation Issues

To date, the majority of breast implant removals have been performed in women with capsular contractures resulting in extremely hard, painful breasts. Women with a diagnosis of silicone-associated connective tissue disease are now facing explantation decisions more frequently than ever before.

Explantation surgery generally takes from one to three hours if the implant has not ruptured, and can usually be done on an outpatient basis. Surgically related complications should in most cases be minor, although there may be bleeding, infection, and skin loss. If silicone has escaped from the implant through slow leakage, bleeding, or outright rupture, the surgery can be difficult—even more so if granulomas have formed. Removal of silicone gel that has escaped into surrounding tissue should be done as soon as it is detected; yet the gel is extremely hard to retrieve completely. When gel has leaked into tissue, the surgeon may opt first to dissect around the capsule in order to gather and clear as much silicone from surrounding tissues as possible. The capsule and implant may then be explanted intact, together, where possible. While this helps to clean out much of the escaped silicone, it also carries with it the necessity of surgically removing more breast tissue, and is a longer and more difficult procedure.

Further, there is currently no known way to remove silicone that has entered the lymphatic system. Foam-coated implants, which may have become thoroughly interwoven with breast tissue, are even harder and more expensive to remove fully.

The implications of surgery are enormous. The information presented here is aimed at enabling a woman to ask the questions she needs honest answers to in order to make one of the most difficult and important decisions of her life. Open dialogue with your surgeon and other physicians is the best means of making the choices that are right for you and your health.

Appendix B

Where to Get Information and Help

Command Trust Network
256 South Linden Drive
Beverly Hills, CA 90212

The CTN provides education and support for women with implants. For information, send $2 and SASE.

National Women's Health Network
1325 G Street, N.W.
Washington, DC 20005
202-347-1140

The National Women's Health Network addresses a broad range of women's health issues.

Public Citizens Health Research Group
2000 P Street, N.W.
Washington, DC 20036
202-833-3000

Public Citizen is a national organization devoted to consumer issues. Its involvement with silicone implants is to petition the FDA, provide consumers with medical and legal information, testify before Congress and the FDA, and make the government, medical, and legal communities, as well as the general public, aware of the problems associated with implants.

Boston Women's Health Book Collective
P.O. Box 192
West Somerville, MA 02144
617-625-0271 Help Line

Information and education regarding women's health issues.

National Association of Silicone Survivors (AS-IS)
Janet Van Winkle
1288 Cork Elm Drive
Kirkwood, MO 63122
314-821-0115

Provides newsletter to members.

Breast Implant Information Foundation
Marie Walsh
25301 Barents Street
Laguna Hills, CA 92653
714-830-2433 (Hotline)

Offers education and support for women with implants.
Coalition of Silicone Survivors

Linda Roth
P.O. Box 129
Broomfield, CO 80038-0129
303-469-8242
303-466-4084 (Fax)

Distributes information and provides education to women afflicted with silicone implant disease.

Children Afflicted by Toxic Substances
Jama Rosanna
60 Oser Avenue
Suite 1
Hauppauge, NY 11788
516-757-6901
800-CATS-199

Seeks to study the effect upon children who have been exposed to second-generation toxic substances such as silicone from breast implants.

Silicone Scene
1050 Cinnamon Lane
Corona, CA 91720
909-737-7769
909-272-1128 (Fax)

Provides information, education and support. For information and a sample copy of newsletter, send $4 and SASE.

800 Numbers

National Registry
800-892-9211

Implant registration and tracking. Manufacturer information updates for registrants.

Food and Drug Administration
800-532-4440
Call for information about FDA policy regarding implants.

Reach to Recovery
American Cancer Society
800-ACS-2345

Physicians' Groups

American Academy of Cosmetic Surgery
159 East Live Oak Avenue
Suite 204
Arcadia, CA 91006
800-221-9808

American Society of Plastic and Reconstructive Surgeons
444 East Algonquin Road
Arlington Heights, IL 60005
800-635-0635

Breast Implant Manufacturers

Baxter Healthcare Corporation
1 Baxter Parkway
Deerfield, IL 60015
800-323-4533

Bioplasty, Inc.
623 Hoover Street N.E.
Minneapolis, MN 55413
612-378-1180

Dow Corning Corporation
P.O. Box 994
Midland, MI 48686-0994
800-442-5442

McGhan Medical Inc.
700 Ward Drive
Santa Barbara, CA 93111
(Note: Inquiries may be made by faxing to 805-967-5839, or writing
to the company in care of the Department of Consumer Affairs.)

Mentor
5425 Hollister Avenue
Santa Barbara, CA 93111
800-525-6747

Porex Technologies
500 Bohannon Road
Fairburn, GA 30213
800-241-0195

Surgitek
3037 Mt. Pleasant Street
Racine, WI 53404
800-634-4397

Cox-Uphoff (CUI Corporation)
1160 Mark Avenue
Carpinteria, CA 93013
800-872-4749

Government Agencies

Arthritis Foundation
P.O. Box 19000
Atlanta, GA 30326
800-283-7800

Food and Drug Administration
Breast Implant Information
HFE-88 5600 Fishers Lane
Rockville, MD 20857
301-443-3170

Lupus Foundation of America
4 Research Place
Suite 180
Rockville, MD 20850
800-558-0121, 301-670-9292

Scleroderma Information

Scleroderma Federation
Peabody Office Building
1 Newbury Street
Peabody, MA 01960
508-535-6600

Notes

1. E. Rosenthal, "Her Ideal of His Ideal, in a Faulty Mirror," *New York Times*, July 22, 1992, p. C12.

2. L. Williams, "Women's Image in a Mirror: Who Defines What She Sees?" *New York Times*, February 6, 1992, p. A1.

3. *Ibid.*

4. *Ibid.*, p. B7.

5. *Ibid.*

6. *Ibid.*

7. Koch, "Augmentation Mammoplasty," *American Journal of Nursing* (1980) 80:1,480.

8. Y. Kumagai, C. Abe, and Y. Shiokawa: "Scleroderma After Cosmetic Surgery. Four Cases of Human Adjuvant Disease," *Arthritis & Rheumatism* 22 (1979): 532-37.

9. Federal Register, FDA, Health & Human Services 56, no. 69 (1991):14620-27.

10. B. F. Uretsky, J. J. O'Brien, E. H. Courtiss, et al., "Augmentation Mammoplasty Associated with a Severe Systemic Reaction," *Annals of Plastic Surgery* 3 (1979):445-47.

11. Y. Kumagai, Y. Shiokawa, T. Medsger, et al., "Clinical Spectrum of Connective Tissue Disease After Cosmetic Surgery," Observations on Eighteen Patients and a Review of the Japanese Literature, *Arthritis & Rheumatism* 27 (1984):1-12.

12. Ad in *Tampa Tribune*, November 12, 1991.

13. FDA Talk Paper, T91-79, December 31, 1991; FDA Warning Letter, December 30, 1991; Barnaby J. Feder, "Dow Corning's Failure in Public Opinion Test," *New York Times*, January 29, 1992, p. D2.

14. Promotional packet sent by the ASPRS in response to telephone queries, as reported in information provided by the National Women's Health Network, November 1992.

15. Nir Kossovsky, M.D., Special Topics Educational Program of the American Society of Clinical Pathologists, Special Topics, No. ST 92-2 (ST-180) (1992) 29, no. 2, N-1 Issn-1056-5981.

16. Evaluation of the Liver Microsomal Enzyme Induction Potential of D-5, Project Report, August 17, 1989, submitted to Dow Corning, on file.

17. Philip S. Hilts, "Strange History of Silicone Held Many Warning Signs," *New York Times*, January 18, 1992, p. A1.

18. M. H. Weisman, T. R. Vecchione, D. Albert, et al., "Connective Tissue Disease Following Breast Augmentation, Preliminary Test of Human Disease Hypothesis," *Journal of Plastic and Reconstructive Surgery* 82 (1988): 626-30.

19. H. Spiera, "Scleroderma After Silicone Augmentation Mammoplasty," *Journal of the American Medical Association* 260 (1988):236-38.

20. L. A. Love, S. R. Weiner, F. B. Vasey, et al., Clinical and Immune Genetic Features of Women Who Develop Myosins After Silicone Implants (MASI), *Arthritis & Rheumatism* 35 (1992):S46.

21. B. Freundlich, J. Tomaszewski, and P. Callegari, "A Sjogren-like Syndrome in Women with Silicone Gel Breast Implants," *Arthritis & Rheumatism* 35 (1992):S67.

22. B. Ostermeyer-Shoaib, B. Patten, and T. Ashizawa, "Motor Neuron Disease After Silicone Breast Implants and Silicone Injections into Face," abstract submitted to The American Neurological Association, August 27, 1992.

23. Hilts, "Strange History of Silicone."

24. Thomas M. Burton, "How Industrial Foam Came to Be Employed in Breast Implants," *Wall Street Journal*, March 25, 1992, p. A1.

25. Memo entitled "Analysis of Dow Corning Data Regarding Carcinogenicity of Silicone Gels," from Acting Chief, Health Sciences Branch, Center for Devices and Radiological Health, FDA, Dr. M. E. Stratmeyer, August 9, 1988, as detailed in a November 9, 1988, Public Citizen letter to Frank Young, former Commissioner of the FDA.

26. Sidney M. Wolfe, M.D., Director, Public Citizen Health Research Group, in a letter to Frank Young, M.D., Ph.D., former Commissioner of the FDA, November 9, 1988, on file.

27. Hans Berkel, M.D., Dale Birdsell, M.D., and Heather Jenkins, M.D., "A Risk Factor for Breast Cancer?" *New England Journal of Medicine* 326 (1992): 1649-1653.

28. U.S. District Court for the District of Columbia, Civil Action No. 89-0391, November 26, 1991, p. 1.

29. Dow Corning internal report, produced in *Cardinal v. Dow Corning Corp.*, on file.

30. Dow Corning internal memo, on file.

31. FDA report, prepared for General and Plastic Surgery Device Panel, 1990, on file.

32. Dow Corning memos from February 19, 1975; February 28, 1975; March 7, 1975; March 14, 1975; March 21, 1975. Produced in *Cardinal v. Dow Corning Corp.*, on file, and FDA report, *ibid.*

33. Dow Corning memos from January 23, 1976; March 19, 1976; May 17, 1976; June 8, 1976. Produced in *Cardinal v. Dow Corning Corp.*, on file.

34. Dow Corning memo from May 13, 1976, produced in *Cardinal v. Dow Corning Corp.*, on file.

35. Dow Corning memo from May 16, 1976, produced in *Cardinal v. Dow Corning Corp.*, on file.

36. P. Hilts, "Maker of Implants Balked at Testing, Its Records Show," *New York Times*, January 13, 1992, p. A1.

37. Dow Corning "interim report," March 6, 1975, on file.

38. Hilts, "Maker of Implants."

39. *Ibid*.

40. P. Hilts, "FDA Seeks Halt in Breast Implants Made of Silicone," *New York Times*, January 7, 1992, p. A1.

41. Dow Corning "Proposal for Development of the Implantable Gel" memo, March 16, 1978, produced in *Cardinal v. Dow Corning Corp.*, on file; and Dow Corning Biological Evaluation of Implantable Silicone Gel report, May 17, 1978, on file.

42. Hilts, "Maker of Implants," p. C5.

43. Dow Corning internal memo, January 15, 1976, produced in *Cardinal v. Dow Corning Corp.*, on file.

44. Dow Corning internal memo, May 17, 1976, on file.

45. T. Smart, "This Man Sounded the Silicone Alarm—in 1976," *Business Week*, January 27, 1992, p. 34.

46. *Ibid*.

47. Dow Corning internal memo, March 31, 1977, on file.

48. *Ibid*.

49. Dow Corning internal memo, September 23, 1983, on file.

50. Dow Corning internal memo, April 29, 1980; September 23, 1981, letter; May 14, 1982, letter; produced in *Cardinal v. Dow Corning Corp.*, on file.

51. *Ibid*.

52. T. Smart, "Breast Implants: What Did the Industry Know, and When?" *Business Week*, January 27, 1992, p. 35.

53. T. Burton and S. McMurray, "Dow Corning Still Keeps Implant Data from Public, Despite Vow of Openness," *Wall Street Journal*, February 18, 1992, p. B3.

54. *Ibid.*

55. Dow Corning internal memo, January 8, 1985, produced in *Cardinal v. Dow Corning Corp.*, on file; and Dow Corning, "Two Year Studies with Miniature Silastic Mammary Implants," report reference 155, April 20, 1970, on file.

56. Hilts, "Maker of Implants."

57. P. Hilts, "Maker of Silicone Breast Implants Says Data Show Them to Be Safe," *New York Times*, January 14, 1992, p. A1.

58. Talk Paper #T91-79, Food and Drug Administration, December 31, 1991.

59. "Breast Implant Hot Line Disconnected," *Tampa Tribune*, January 1, 1992.

60. Burton and McMurray, "Dow Corning Still Keeps Implant Data."

61. P. Hilts, "Biggest Maker of Breast Implants Is Said to Be Abandoning Market," *New York Times*, March 19, 1992, p. A1.

62. A. Eagan, *New Woman*, July 1992, p. 123.

63. T. Burton, "How Industrial Foam Came to Be Employed in Breast Implants," *Wall Street Journal*, March 25, 1992, p. A1.

64. *Ibid.*

65. *Ibid.*

66. *Ibid.*

67. *Ibid.*

68. FDA Backgrounder #BG 91-6.1, August 1991.

69. Burton, "How Industrial Foam Came to Be Employed in Breast Implants."

70. S. Blakeslee, "The True Story Behind Breast Implants," *Glamour*, August 1991, p. 186.

71. Burton, "How Industrial Foam Came to Be Employed in Breast Implants."

72. M. Wald, "An Ex-Chemist's Formula for Dow Corning," *New York Times*, February 19, 1992, p. D1.

73. Public Citizen letter #1 143, November 9, 1988, on file.

74. Public Citizen letter #1 177, August 3, 1989, on file.

75. U.S. District for the District of Columbia, Civil Action No. 89-0391, November 26, 1991, p. 1.

76. T. Lewin, "As Silicone Issue Grows, Women Take Agony and Anger to Court," *New York Times*, January 19, 1992, p. A1.

77. FDA report, prepared for General and Plastic Surgery Device Panel, 1991, on file.

78. Hearing Before the Human Resources and Intergovernmental Relations Subcommittee of the Committee on Government Operations, "Is the FDA Protecting Patients from the Dangers of Silicone Breast Implants," December 18, 1990, p. 1.

79. Blakeslee, "The True Story Behind Breast Implants."

80. FDA report, prepared for General and Plastic Surgery Device Panel, 1991, on file.

81. Department of Health and Human Services, Docket # 91N-0372, September 20, 1991.

82. P. Hilts, "FDA Seeks Halt in Breast Implants Made of Silicone," *New York Times*, January 7, 1992, p. A1.

83. E. Rosenthal, "Her Image of His Ideal, in a Faulty Mirror," *New York Times*, July 22, 1992, p. C2.

84. Nicholas Regush, "Toxic Breasts," *Mother Jones*, January/February 1992, pp. 25-31.

85. "Silicone Breast Implants," Women's Health Coalition, 1990, p. 1.

86. Philip J. Hilts, "Women Lobby for Freedom to Choose Breast Implants," *Minneapolis Star Tribune*, October 21, 1991, p. 5A.

87. Joan E. Rigdon, "Informed Consent?" *Wall Street Journal*, March 12, 1992, p. A1.

88. *Ibid.*, p. A4.

89. Hilts, "Women Lobby for Freedom."

90. Susan Kissir, "Beauty and the Breast," *Health Watch*, July/August 1991, p. 43.

91. William Carter, L. William Luria, et al., "Silicone Singled Out for Only Breast Implants," *Tampa Tribune*, January 19, 1992, p. 2. (Commentary).

92. Rigdon, "Informed Consent?"

93. Carole Tarrant, "Manufacturers, Surgeons Defend Breast Implants," *Tampa Tribune-Times*, April 21, 1991, p. 1.

94. Rigdon, "Informed Consent?"

95. Regush, "Toxic Breasts," p. 28.

96. Felicity Barringer, "Surgeons Accuse F.D.A. of Creating Panic on Implants," *New York Times*, January 16, 1992, p. B9.

97. A. Eagan, *New Woman*, July 1992, p. 123.

98. Marilyn Elias, "Benefits of Implant Removal," *USA Today*, October 13, 1992, p. 1D.

99. F. M. Wigley, R. Miller, M. C. Hochberg, et al., "Augmentation Mammoplasty in Patients with Systems Sclerosis." Data from the Baltimore Scleroderma Research Center and Pittsburgh Scleroderma Data Bank, *Arthritis & Rheumatism* 35 (1992):S46.

100. C. E. Dugowson, J. Daling, T. D. Koepsell, et al., "Silicone Breast Implants and Risk for RA," *Arthritis & Rheumatism* 35 (1992):S66.

101. J. A. Goldman, S. H. Lamm, and L. C. Cooper, "Breast Implants Are Not Associated with an Excess of Connective Tissue Disease" (ctd), *Arthritis & Rheumatism* 35 (1992):S65.

102. R. M. Goldblum, R. P. Relley, A. A. O'Donnell, D. Pyron, and J. P. Heggers, "Antibodies to Silicone Elastomers and Reactions to Ventriculoperitoneal Shunts," *Lancet* 340 (1992):510-13.

103. Rigdon, "Informed Consent?"

104. *Ibid*.

Glossary

Adjuvant. A substance which increases immune response.

Antibody. A protein produced by the immune system which reacts with a specific antigen.

Antigen. A substance capable of inducing the immune system to produce an antibody.

Antinuclear antibody. An antibody directed against the nucleus of cells. This antibody is present in the blood of almost all patients with Systemic Lupus Erythematosis, but is also found in many other conditions.

Autoimmune. Immune system attack upon the body's own tissues (see also immune system).

Biopsy. The removal of tissue from the living body in order to examine it both grossly and under the microscope.

Breast implant. Silicone material inserted into or under the tissue of the breast. The types include: single lumen with a silicone/silica envelope and silicone gel interior; double lumen with a gel portion and saline portion; and a polyurethane coated silicone implant.

Capsular contracture. The fibrous tissue that forms around the breast implant.

Connective tissue. The structures which bind together and support the body. These include tendons, ligaments, joints, bones, cartilage and synovium (joint lining).

Electron microscope. A microscope in which an electron beam, instead of light, forms an image. This permits greater magnification than a traditional light microscope.

Envelope. An encompassing structure or membrane such as the outer layer of a breast implant.

Epidemiology. The study of the relationship of factors determining the frequency and distribution of human disease.

Gel. A glue-like material in breast implants composed of small repeating units of silicon; oxygen end blocked with methyl groups.

Human adjuvant disease. An early term used to indicate the connective tissue diseases occurring in women with breast implants.

Inert. Having no action; not reacting with the body.

Immune system. The body's complex system for distinguishing foreign material from itself and neutralizing, metabolizing, and eliminating that which is foreign. It is composed both of cells (macrophages, lymphocytes, neutrophils and protein antibodies) in tissues and in blood.

Immunogen. A substance capable of inducing an immune response.

Lumen. The cavity of a breast implant which may be single-filled with saline or silicone gel or double-filled with one of each.

Lymphocyte. A white cell with a single nucleus found in the blood, lymphatic system, and in tissue, with the capability to kill tumor cells and transplanted tissues, as well as to produce antibodies.

Macrophage. An amoeba-like white cell with a single nucleus, which wanders through the body's tissue ingesting and metabolizing foreign material.

Neutrophil. A white cell with a multi-lobed nucleus which ingests and metabolizes foreign material while being the predominant white cell in blood.

Pathology. The speciality of medicine that studies structural and functional changes in tissues and organs.

Prosthesis. An artificial substitute for a missing body part.

Polydimethylsiloxane. The chemical name for the polymer called silicone.

Polymer. A natural or synthetic chemical compound consisting of repeating structural units.

Polyurethane. The polymer with an -NH COO- linkage that is a foam placed around some breast implants.

Saline. Salt water which forms the interior material of saline filled silicone envelope implants.

Silicone. An organic compound in which some or all of the carbon has been replaced by silicon.

Silicon. A non metallic light element with the atomic number 14.

Silica. Silicone dioxide which is a component of the breast implant envelope and a known immunogen when inhaled.

Silicone associated connective tissue disease. The typical rheumatic conditions occurring in women with breast implants.

Synovium. The joint lining which produces joint fluid.

Systemic. Affecting the body as a whole.

Index

147

Explantation. *See* Implant removal (explantation)
Eyes, dry, 25, 32

F

Fatigue, 23, 25, 33-34, 41
importance of seeking care for, 105
FDA (Food and Drug Administration), 1, 7, 16, 29, 59-88, 117, 119, 133, 134
approval process, bypassing of, 76-77
assurances of safety, areas of, list of, 17
cancer concerns, 39, 77-78
claim that safety data was incomplete (November 1991), 83-84
conference on silicone in medical devices (February, 1991), 82
designation of implants as "unproven" (Class III rating), 18-19, 76, 79, 100
Dow Corning, warning letter to (December, 1991), 20
Dow Corning's communication controversy, 72-73
early test results, 67-68
educational pamphlets, 97
foam implants, 36, 39, 74, 77-78
gel reformulation, 64-67
General and Plastic Surgery Devices Panel of, 17, 75, 79-81, 83-84, 95
genetic markers, 28
"grandfather" designation, 77
hotline, 85
injectable silicone, 95
"lack of testing" abuses, aired in courtrooms, 71-72
limited powers of, 78-80
listing of autoimmune disease as a possible "significant risk," 80
lung disease, reports of, 32
making of the "silicone safety case," 92

MDR (Medical Device Reporting) Program, 19-20
moratorium (1992), 2, 16-17, 19, 84-85, 86, 95-96, 107
National Implant Registry, 37, 84, 132
plastic surgeons in private practice, attitude of, 92-93
PMAs (Pre-market Approval) applications, 79, 80, 82-83
product literature from manufacturers, 19-20
Representative Weiss's actions, 71-72, 80-82
risk information, requirement of more accurate, 83
roadblocks to recognizing silicone-induced disease, summary of, 75
silicone gel vs. saline gel implants, studies comparing, 42
Teich v. FDA and Dow Corning, 63
Feldene, 43
Feng, Lu-Jean, 99
Fetuses, 40-41
Fever
low-grade, 25, 55, 125
Fibrocystic breast disease, 15
Fibromyalgia (fibrosistis), 23-24, 57-58
Fibrosis, 30, 69
Fisher, Jack, 96
Food and Drug Research Laboratories, 71
Foreign studies, 18, 19
Freundlich, Bruce, 32

G

Gastrointestinal symptoms, 25
Genetics, 37-38, 50
Gerow, Frank, 16
Gershwin, Eric, 24
Glamour, 74
Golden, Kristen, 5
Goldrich, Sybil, 79
Government Operations Committees, 71

"Grandfather" statute (medical device law statute), 17, 19, 77
Grant, Cary, 104
Granulomas, 29
Griffiths, Edward, 74

H

Harrison, Myron, 88
Hayes, Dan T., 69
Health Care Business, 67
Health insurance, 44-45, 78, 113-14, 117, 123
Heart disease, 45
Heggers, John Paul, 30, 99
Helen (case study), 45-46
Helper T cells, 53
  definition of, 59-60
Hematomas, 108, 125
Heredity, 37-38, 50
Heyer-Schulte Corporation, 73
Hippocratic oath, 100
Histamines, 54
H. L. Moffitt Cancer Center, 98
Hopkins, Mariann, 72
Hotline
  Dow Corning, 20, 72-73
  FDA, 85
House Oversight and Investigations Subcommittee, 76
Human Genome Project, 37
Hyperplasia, 33
Hypertension, 12

I

Immune system, 6, 20, 24, 33, 47-59
  breast implants as infection "allies," 39
  implant removal, 110
  lack of safety assurances regarding, FDA opinion on, 17
  operation of, four basic stages of, 50
  patient predispositions to silicone disease, 37-38
  product claims of safety, 70-71

responses to other silicone implants, 35
silica as an immunogen, 28
types of immunity, 50
Immunization, 50
Immunogens, 28
Implant removal (explantation), 1-3, 41-44, 47-48
  costs of, 72-73, 107, 109, 113-14
  disfigurement, 108-9
  Dow funding of, 72-73
  improved health post-operatively, 12, 34, 85, 109-10, 114, 118
  loss of positive self-image, 110-13
  loss of sensitivity, 109
  opting for, 114-15
  overview of, 122-30
  reactions by mates, 111-13
  resistance from surgeons, 111
  risks of surgery, 108
  silicone migration and leakage, 34, 107, 110, 129-30
  TRAM flap procedures, 109, 129
Implant ruptures, 17, 118
  "silent," 99, 106
  symptoms following, 25
Implants
  silicone, other than breast implants, 7, 35, 40. *See also* Implant removal (explantation); Implant ruptures; Injection procedure
Indocin, 43
Infants, newborn, 40-41
Infection, 39, 125
Inflammation, 55, 67, 125
  chronic, definition of, 54
Information lines. *See* Hotlines
Injection procedure, 16, 95
Insurance, 44-45, 78, 113-14, 117, 123
Interleukins, 52
Irene (case study), 112-13
Iverson, Ronald, 91

J

Jane (case study), 122
Japan, 16, 18, 19, 29

Jefferson Medical College, 82
Johns Hopkins University, 71, 99-
100
Joint implants, 35, 40
Joint pain, 23, 25, 31, 56
*Journal of Plastic and Reconstructive
Surgery*, 30
Joyce (case study), 41-42
Justice Department, 72, 78

K

Katie (case study), 102-3
Kessler, David A., 18, 84-87, 92,
95-96
Killer T cells, 53
definition of, 59-60
Kossovsky, Nir, 28

L

Lancet, 99
La Russa, Don, 90
Laura (case study), 15
Lawsuits, 44, 74
lack of testing abuses, 70-72
reluctance to pursue, 79
Teich v. FDA and Dow Corning,
63
Leakage. *See* Silicone migration and
leakage
LeVier, Robert R., 68, 69, 70
Lip enhancement, 16
Liquid silicone, 16, 95
Lou Gehrig's disease, 34, 58
Love, Lucy, 32
Lumpectomies, 107
Lung diseases, 26, 37, 55
basic description of, 32
hazards of silicone exposure, 28
Lupus, 13
ANA tests, 24
erythemtosus, systemic, 31, 56-57
symptoms of, 24. *See also*
Rheumatic diseases
Luria, William, 92
Lymph nodes, 11, 15
basic description of, 33

lymphatic systems, overview of,
55
swollen lymph nodes (lymphadenopathy), 24, 25, 31, 52-
53, 56
Lymphocytes, 54, 55
definition of, 59

M

McGhan Medical Corporation, 73,
83, 96, 128, 133
McKennon, Keith, 88
Macrophages, 28, 29-30, 32
basic description of, 59-60
chronic inflammation, 54
conglomeration of, around
silicone, 52-53
Mammograms, 22, 85, 87, 99, 108
basic description of, 106-7
TRAM flap procedures, 109
Margo (case study), 42
Markham, Harold, 73, 74
Maryland, regulations in, 97
Mast cells, 54
Mastectomies, 2, 22, 31, 73, 89-90,
107, 110, 112
MDR (Medical Device Reporting)
Program, 19-20
Medical Devices Bulletin, 17
Medical device law statute ("grand-
father" statute), 17, 19
Medic Alert, 37
Medicare, 78
Medsger, Tom, 19
Memory loss, 25
Mentor Corporation, 72, 83, 128,
134
Menstruation, 45, 105
Migration. *See* Silicone migration
and leakage
Miller, Fred, 28, 32
Minneapolis Star Tribune, 91
Monocytes, 59
Mother Jones, 90
Motrin, 43
Mouth, dry, 25, 32
MRI (magnetic resonance imaging),
107

151

Rose, Noel R., 99
Rudy, James, 73, 100
Ruptures, implant. *See* Implant
    ruptures
Rylee, Robert T., 67-68, 70, 85

S

St. Petersburg Medical Clinic, 43
Salisbury, Tom, 66-68
Scarring, 55, 108, 127
Scleritis, 56
Scleroderma, 13, 18, 32, 57. *See
    also* Rheumatic diseases
Scleroderma Foundation, 32
Scotfoam Corporation, 74
Scott Industrial Foam, 74
Sedimentation rates, 26
Self-image, 3, 90, 117, 123, 124
    cultural pressures for "perfection,"
        1, 2-3, 5-6
    implant removal, 110-11. *See also*
        Psychological issues
Sexuality, 26, 41-42, 110
Shaw, William, 34, 98
Shell-destruction/erosion hypothe-
    sis, 28, 52
Silica, 27-28
Silicone devices
    other than breast implants, 7, 35,
        40
Silicone migration and leakage, 17,
    51-52, 88
    basic description of, 22-23, 38, 52
    Dow's product claims of safety,
        66, 68, 69
    foreign studies on, 18
    "gel-bleed phenomenon," 22,
        30, 40, 66, 68, 88, 118
    implant removal, 34, 107, 110,
        129-30
    shell-destruction/erosion hypothe-
        sis, 28, 52
Silver, Richard, 24
Silverstein, Melvin, 100
Simethicone, 7
Sinus irritation, 26
Sjogren's Syndrome, 32

Skin necrosis, 126
Skin tightening, 26
Sleep patterns, 23, 24
Smoking, 35, 37, 87
Spiera, Harry, 32
Splenomegaly, 56
Sporkin, Stanley, 63, 78
Sports, 23
Squibb, 73, 74
Subpoena power, 78
Suicide, 16, 26, 110
Surgery. *See* Implant removal
    (explantation); Mastectomies;
    Reconstructive surgery
Surgitek, 74
Systemic lupus Erythematosus
    (SLE), 31

T

Talcott, Tom, 66-69, 73
Tampa Tribune, 92
T cells, 53, 59-60, 99
TDA (2-toluene diamine), 36, 75,
    81-82
Teich v. FDA and Dow Corning, 63
Thalidomide, 45, 77
Theodur, 11
Thompson, J. Kevin, 5
Toxic porphyria, 26-27
TRAM flap procedure, 109, 129
Transsexuals, 29
Trapezius muscle, 54-55
Tumors, 15, 17. *See also*
    Mammograms

U

Ultrasound tests, 106
University of California at Davis, 24
University of California at Los
    Angeles (UCLA), 28, 34, 98
University of California at San
    Diego, 30
University of Florida, Gainesville,
    96
University of South Florida (USF),
    Department of Rheumatology,
        6, 15, 19, 21, 31, 35, 93